Love Yourself Fit®

Lisa Nordquist

www.LoveYourselfFit.com

ISBN 978-0-9915347-2-2

Publication Date: January 2015

Published by Lisa Nordquist, San Diego, CA
www.loveyourselffit.com

 Written by Lisa Nordquist, www.LoveYourselfFit.com
 Edited by Andrea Susan Glass, www.WritersWay.com
 Interior Design by Aaron Salts, aaronsalts@yahoo.com
 Sharina Menke, MainKeyMedia.com
 Cover Design by Derek Murphy, www.CreativIndieCovers.com

Printed in the United States of America

For Gillian & Camryn

I wish you both the true love of your whole selves.

You are miraculous! I love you all the way.

Mommy

With Appreciation

I'd like to thank my husband, Doug, and my Mom for your unending support, coaching and encouragement with this project. My Dad and lovely little girls, thanks for your patience and sweet words. You have each been part of this book becoming a reality. My extended family, author grandmas, and brother, Nick-the-video-God, for assistance as needed. Gary Rush, Felisha English, Kristen Miner, and my many other friends for being sounding boards, cheerleaders, or coaches along the way. All the great teachers, who are too many to name, for your wisdom through the ages and gifts you've given us. Jacob Glass, for helping me to understand the Course and the meaning of so many principles. Sharina Menke and Alan Hays for the masterful artwork and Jasen Miner for the gorgeous photos. I'd like to thank my editor, Andrea Glass, for her extended guidance and advice, and also Anne Geiberger and Lora Van Renselaar—you each helped me clarify the message. Designer Derek Murphy for the cover, patience and advice. Michele Baker for her marketing expertise.

TABLE OF CONTENTS

At your core you are spirit.

You are more than a collection of cells, bones, and organs.
Yet, when it comes to fitness or weight loss,
you believe yourself to be a corporeal mass of muscle
tissue and digestive processes. Fitness, without reverence for
what you are, will remain an empty and fruitless pursuit.

Lisa Nordquist

INTRODUCTION

I grew up in sunny, surfer girl infested San Diego County. From childhood I struggled with my body, weight, and food—physically and mentally. As the child of an NFL player—dark haired, light skinned—and of Scandinavian descent, I wasn't the waify sun-kissed California type. Although, when that Beach Boys song played, I would pretend they were including us large-legged, ivory gals in their dreamy descriptions. I always remember feeling awkward in my own skin, not being athletic, and noticing my size compared to other little surfer girls. At the same time, I would overeat after school and always try to swindle dessert after meals. As puberty descended, so did feminine curves, and I promptly declared war on my body.

This war would last well into adulthood. It started as most wars do—a disagreement between two parties that spirals into a crevice of cruelty and attack. My body wanted to be the dark-haired, larger-build Scandinavian girl, and I wanted it to be the cute little blond surfer girl. We fought about it again and again, and I'd lose every time.

The battles were long and ugly. Sometimes starving and strange diets, other times brutal exercise regimens followed by extended periods of couch surfing. I always entered the battlegrounds with a sense of desperation, dissatisfaction, and not "good enough-ness"—the opposite of what I really wanted. I wanted to love my looks, feel good in my body, and somehow have this fitness food thing be easy, or at least organic to me. I was always trying to win the war, and I was encouraged to keep fighting by my culture and fellow ladies-in-arms. Food and my body became the enemy, thinness and beauty my would-be victory.

Nothing I tried worked to get me moving or eating well for long. When I went off to college, the war escalated and so did my disappointment and frustration. I studied psychology and developed an interest in psychosomatics—how state of mind affects the body and vice versa. It wasn't long after I graduated that I decided to solve my body problems for good by becoming professionally obsessed: I entered the fitness industry.

In the industry I gained material knowledge and yet I continued to lament. I knew what to physically do, but I still struggled mentally and behaviorally. When I consistently practiced the right behaviors, I didn't feel any better about my body, or fall in love with fitness. I still didn't love exercise or my body and I fought with food. Being in the business, I felt more pressure than ever to look fit, and no matter how fit I became it still wasn't enough. There was always a higher level to reach and no real love—for body, food, or exercise.

I soon realized my clients were dealing with the same problem—and lack of a real solution—that I was. I could give them the physical prescriptions for fitness or weight loss, but I could do little to help them maintain those behaviors independently and consistently. Nor did I have anything to offer that would help them fall in love with fitness or their bodies. Even when they reached their physical goals, the same judgmental mind-state remained. There was no long-term psychologically healthy way of being with food or relating to their bodies. There was no love. We had simply created a conditional relationship: numerical conditions to be met, conditional adherence, and self-love and approval based on conditions. The fitness programs we created reminded me of a marriage for money: it was conditional and based on superficial results.

This ongoing struggle led me to seek answers in somewhat uncharted fitness waters: within. And I don't mean taking a deep breath and calling it mind-body fitness. I mean the nitty-gritty area of feelings, thoughts, beliefs, source of habits, and the psycho-emotional triggers of behavior.

You know what I'm talking about: *the places you don't really want to go.* I began to investigate and explore the areas of my mind and emotions that were dictating or affecting my behaviors. As I focused inward I realized that most of my everyday choices were not coming from what I logically knew about fitness and nutrition, but from my state of mind, feelings, relationships, self-concept, and the whole spectrum of my life. An unsatisfying day at work or a fight with a boyfriend would lead to craving dessert—looking for fulfillment I didn't have in another area of my life. I saw my choices about food and exercise radically intertwined with what was happening in my heart, mind, relationships, work, family, finances, and sense of spiritual connection.

I had been involved in New Thought since I was a child. My parents would take me to watch Terry Cole-Whittaker at the ripe old age of seven, and throughout my life I returned to study similar spiritual principles. I knew these principles worked. I had seen it in my own life and in the lives of others. The aligned mind is powerful. I eventually realized I could weave these thought principles into a new way of relating to my body and fitness. I set out to create a new mindset to bridge the gap between knowing what I should do and doing it *consistently.* And I wanted so badly to love my body, really love it without conditions. Over time the dysfunctional relationship I had with my body, food, and self-care dissolved and a new one emerged; I found my love of exercise and peace with food.

As I grew into this new self-care (fitness) mindset, I began to feel I was doing a disservice to my personal training clients. They were all coming to me for the magic weight loss recipe and were convinced it was hidden somewhere under the elliptical machine. Though client after client believed all she needed was to find the right abdominal exercise or calorie-free cracker, I knew each one needed a shift in mindset. Through traditional means I could only offer them a temporary external fix or babysit them through a workout. What they needed was a thought process that could help them actually choose better—a balance between the white flag of the couch and DEFCON 2 at the gym. And I knew the wall separating body-mind-spirit-life had to come down. Conditional approaches based in separateness, judgment, and avoidance were not the answers. They needed what I was growing into with my self-care: a real connection with my body and feeling good in the everyday practice of self-care. I knew that once they had this relationship established, the physical elements of weight loss and fitness would follow and stick.

And so I wrote this book. My intention with the "Love Yourself Fit®" movement is to help those who are at war with their bodies, food, and exercise to declare peace. If you are one of those soldiers, I want you to put down your magazines of ammunition (pun intended) and diet revolvers and sit down for peace talks with your body. Hear what I, your arbitrator, have to say and what your body is telling you, and then decide if you want love or war.

I want you to experience such peace with your body that you can move on to the really meaningful elements of your life and make amazing contributions to the planet. Considering all that is happening in our world today, proportionately your cellulite isn't that important and likely doesn't need the energy you're giving it.

I imagine an evolution of energy expenditure for our culture. If women would take half of the energy, money, and time we spend on our bodies and looks, obsessing, dressing, and "fixing" ourselves and channel it toward things like medical research, learning and educating, feeding the hungry, or running the government efficiently, we would rapidly change our world for the better. Furthermore, your daughter, granddaughter, niece, or neighbor's kid would be free of this jaded feminine legacy. The little girls behind you could move on to more meaningful stuff too. Can you imagine young women on the cover of magazines for solving a super equation or engineering a space station instead of another ode to the best bikini bod? I realize this evolution of our collective mind is big. But so are you and I.

14

I also want to warn you: I use adult language and can be uncomfortably blunt. This book is for grownups, not your twelve year-old daughter. If you are offended, I am so sorry. I also mostly use the word "she" and female examples, because the majority of people interested in this subject are female and this is traditionally a feminine issue—not because I believe women to be victims of "he" in published works. If you are offended by this, I am so sorry. I will also suggest you start moving your body and peer into your own psycho-emotional world. I do not believe the majority need professional guidance to do either one of these things, but if you think you may be at risk for going bat-shit crazy or having a coronary event, you are grown up enough to know better and should seek professional guidance along either of these areas. You are responsible for your own thoughts, actions, and choices.

Keep in mind as you read that the "Love Yourself Fit®" philosophy can be used in conjunction with any physical program or book. Most fitness books and practitioners talk exclusively about the physical environment and elements required for good self-care. I don't. If you are looking for another diet or work out program, this ain't it! *Love Yourself Fit®* is about creating the internal environment to make fitness a loving, enjoyable daily practice. There are no physical exercises, programs, or recipes here. I will not tell you what to eat or which exercises to do at the gym. This book is a training guide for your mind or a roadmap to a better mindset, not a weight loss quick fix or a gimmick. Your workouts will not be with dumbbells or treadmills, but with your level of self-honesty, emotions, thoughts, beliefs, insight, and habits. The only equipment you'll need is pen, paper, and your own willingness. For where the mind leads, the body will follow.

SECTION I

The Great Divide:

The Real Reason You're Struggling with Weight, Food, & Exercise

CHAPTER 1

The Great Divide:
Stuck in a Dead-End Relationship with Fitness

"Seek not to change the world but choose to change your mind about the world."

A Course in Miracles

If you are like most people trying to get into shape, you are at war. And it's not your first time. In fact, you may be a five-star general you've been fighting your belly fat for so long. You've been to the battlefield before and return this day, scarred and bloodied, to defeat the legion of cellulite that has established new colonies along the back side of your thighs. They have raped your muscles for the last time! Once more you pledge in disgust: "Vegetables and whole grains will be my armor, and exercise will be my sword!" With visions of a bikini clad victory streaming through your head, you declare a fat-crusade, assemble your lard camouflaging workout gear, arm your phone with a calorie counting app, and enlist comrades to join your campaign…tomorrow. "Yes! We ride—the elliptical—at dawn!" you think as you settle in for what could be your last night ever to eat chocolate covered pizza and cheesy

potato crunchies. This time you're doing it; you're getting really serious…
tomorrow. Tonight though, you dine as if it were your last day on earth;
tonight you sit on Diet Row.

You are not the only one condemned to the weight loss war wagon. Our
entire world is at war with adipose tissue. Fat has been declared the enemy
by every entity from elementary schools to retail stores, governments to
your local book club. It seems as though the entire planet has adopted a
contentious approach to bodies, weight loss, exercise, and food—mostly
in an effort to correct an expanding overweight pandemic.

Think about the way we approach fitness and weight loss. We've identified edible good guys and bad guys, established training and boot camps,
strategized label reading and nutrition, and fitness manuals, equipment,
and programs are now "weapons" against fat. Half the food in your kitchen
has been designated E-V-I-L and made out to be a minion of the enemy.
Horror reports fill the airways daily espousing incomplete truths and
projections about the toxic substances you're ingesting. The media dourly
projects the next generation's early demise at the hands of the enemy. Fear,
contempt, and fighting fill your internal and external reality every day in
regards to health and fitness.

As one is recruited or enlists herself in this body blitzkrieg, the accom-
panying antagonistic mindset creates an internal revolt; a mental and
emotional rebellion begins to emerge. Feelings of deprivation and dread,
struggle, and separation surface as you begin to feel the contradiction
within. You judge your body harshly and self-care becomes a chore. Your
regimen mirrors this as a "to-do" list of muscular and digestive chores.
You *should* eat your veggies, you *have* to spend an hour on the treadmill,
and you *must* lose weight. Food is already the enemy, but now numbers
become demi-gods. Any deviation from the doctrine of weight loss is
accompanied by guilt and self-flagellation. The entire endeavor destroys
the possibility of enjoying the process, ruins food, and segregates you

from your body. Your heart, mind, spirit, schedule, relationships, life-style—essentially you—are suddenly null and void, not an important part of getting or staying fit.

To quote Dr. Phil: *How's it working for you?* Has this war been helpful in improving your health, weight, or body image? Have the fearful facts been encouraging? How about the body loathing—has hating your body been inspiring? If you're reading this book, it's likely conventional fitness isn't working for you. Actually, it may be working against you.

Much of what you associate with fitness is negative and uninspiring. The general vibe of weight loss, exercise, and fitness sucks…the energy right out of you. Think about the term "weight loss". What comes to mind? Unicorns and rainbows or "Oh, shit"? The language you use is contrary to what you want. The word "weight" is heavy, big, hard to move and implies great effort. The same with "loss"; it brings up thoughts of suffering, deficit, or emotional pain. If you're beginning a quest for lightness, health, and loving your body, why launch with the vibes of heaviness, difficulty, and loss? All of this punitive, negative crap is adding a climate, or energy of resistance or difficulty, enlarging the weight you want to lose.

Am I saying you can meditate on unicorns and rainbows and still get in shape? I don't know about that. But meditating on just about anything would be more helpful than trying to hate yourself into shape.

In the last four decades the fitness and weight loss movement has imbedded itself in our society. In this time we've become more obsessed with our bodies, weight loss, and food than ever. We've grown increasingly resistant, deconditioned, overweight, guilty, and have developed more extreme, even harmful, methods to rectify the problem. Moreover, we're less kind, healthy, and loving toward our bodies and more judgmental, cruel, and depressed about all bodies. We can't seem to find a way to win the war or stop fighting it once we've started. The worst part is that there's no victory on this battlefield, no end to the fighting with this mindset. In this state, you'll awaken every morning with the same enemies—in your fridge, on the menu, in your closet, and in the mirror.

With a warlike mindset in place, fitness is negative, effortful, and anything but long lasting. And don't forget mean. You get mean. Have you ever met a meaner bitch than the naked one staring back at you in the mirror? I think not. Who would want to live in a state of war, deprivation, and verbal abuse like this every day, particularly with that bitch?

This hate state of being is the opposite of what you really want.

Think about what you want when it comes to your body, eating, and fitness. If you were writing your own story, would you want to write a war biography or a romance novel? *Are you kidding me?* Romance novel all the way! You want to be swept off your feet by some good smelling, hunk-of-a-diet! You want to ride off into the sunset of happily-ever-healthy! Actually, you want to love your body and feel good in it. If you believed it were possible, you'd want to love your fitness program too—actually enjoy the activities and edibles. You don't want to struggle, count, measure, or weigh anything. You want it to be easy and feel like second nature. You want to be healthy and look your best without breaking the time-energy piggy bank.

You know what you want. And you know what you're doing isn't working. *But it should be!* Your inability to maintain the physical behaviors required to sustain a fit body is not because you lack the knowledge; you're perfectly well informed. You have a surplus of resources at your disposal to assist you in learning and practicing healthy behaviors, particularly in the United States. You're offered web sites, magazines, programs, gyms, books, diets, equipment, and professional trainers. The government sponsors health-promoting programs like the 5 A Day Program and the President's Council on Physical Fitness and Sports. Restaurants and food manufacturers have jumped on the bandwagon with heart-healthy and diet-friendly menus, labels, and products. Networks and newspapers include reports on nutrition and exercise-related research on a daily basis. There's a gym, a YMCA, or a yoga studio in every town. Now there are TV shows, YouTube videos, and networks dedicated entirely to weight loss and fitness. And let's not forget the slough of apps that have recently emerged to help anyone track her eating, calories, weight loss, or starvation-induced rage. You have at your disposal more options for achieving and maintaining good health than at any other time in history.

You also have the desire, at least most Americans do. Millions of us want to get fit and we pour our money and hope into any and every fitness trend or weight loss solution on the market. Even though health risks and premature death sometimes loom as consequences if we don't do something different, we still wrestle to change our behavior.

Yet there are those who don't struggle, those who have succeeded as body warriors, fighting the fight without apparent struggle or contradiction. Those who have conquered this battle seem to be an entirely different breed of human: the gym rat, jock, or fitness freak. These are the same human mutations that staff the fitness industry and engineer new exercise products and services for the rest of us. Mutants! Those of us unlucky enough to be born without this fitness chromosome struggle year after year to achieve a reasonable body weight, exercise regularly, and eat healthfully.

Initially we're inclined to assess a fit person's behaviors and try to copy them. In fact, this is what most diet and exercise programs are: a set of behaviors for you to duplicate. Yet you can't duplicate behaviors if the part of your brain in charge of behavior is on strike or out of the loop. Furthermore, these behaviors in and of themselves are only part of successful self-care. What will ultimately work is not some mystical running routine, miracle diet, or impenetrable type of self-discipline. The true source of a fit person's success is her aligned state of mind, emotion, and spirit. She has little or no conflict within. She is crystal clear about her daily intentions of staying fit, eating healthfully, and exercising. It's her inner state of being that creates her long-term success and maintainable behaviors. The daily decision to exercise and eat healthfully is executive: it comes from upstairs, past the taste buds.

When you know better, you'll do better claim the fitness industry, medical community, and nutrition experts. So they keep giving you more information. But knowledge itself doesn't wield enough power to alter one's behavior: knowing doesn't mean doing. Even extremely negative consequences often don't influence a person's decisions. As evolved as we are, humans are not run by logic alone. Nor do we act purely from zoological instincts—the complexities of the mature, intelligent human being overextend the parameters of Behavior Modification. No matter what you feel like before you shave your legs, you're not a chimp!

The "know-do" equation is part of learning and behavior change but likely has fallen short of controlling your behavior when it comes to fried food or dark chocolate. As part of the majority, being informed about health and fitness has not led you to permanently implement the best that science has to offer. All of the resources, desire, knowledge, and role models in the world and you continue to battle overeating, under activity, and overweight.

Why?

Your state of mind is *definitive.* Mind-state determines your outlook on everything from bunnies to your coworkers to politics. Therefore, *it's the way you think about your body, exercise, food, and weight loss that's the primary problem*, not the pork chops or potato chips. It's your lack of internal alignment that interferes with your use of the knowledge, resources, or role models available to you. When you change your thinking about fitness, your mind-state and energy, your behavior will naturally follow suit.

Think about what got you off track last time you were on an exercise or weight loss program. Was there not enough equipment at the gym? A shortage of exercise classes perhaps? Maybe you didn't buy enough carrot sticks or grapefruit to keep you away from the cheese tray or flourless chocolate cake at work. *The truth is it was none of the above!* Your mind wandered, your heart wandered, or you veered off course by way of cognitive choice—a lack of internal mind-body-spirit alignment.

Therefore, you can read four hundred magazines with the super diets or dynamite ab workouts, but until you shift your mindset about your body, exercise, and food you won't move into lasting, easy, and enjoyable self-care. It will still be a war. With a warlike mindset, fitness will only become your lifestyle with force, fighting, and judgment.

Don't believe me? If you awoke delighted with your "ideal" body tomorrow, how long would you be able to maintain it? How long before you overeat or blow off the gym? You don't know how to live in your conceptual "ideal" body—you're not in the mind-state or energy of it—therefore it would be impossible for you to stay there. Fit doesn't exist for you as a cognitive lifestyle or emotional reality yet. It's still under your chore category or on your something–to–conquer list. Or you have some internal resistance, fear, or avoidance program playing in your mental background. If you're struggling with fitness, it's still a destination for you. Energetically, mentally, emotionally, spiritually, physically, and within the reality of your everyday life you're not aligned with a fit state of being.

The Law of Attraction basically states that the focus of your attention becomes more dominant in your life. It makes sense. If you hate spiders, you'll notice them around your house and yard. If you want a boob job, you'll pay attention to every female chest that crosses your path. If you're on a diet, you'll want every bite of food you're not allowed to eat, and then some! In other words, you expand in your awareness that which you focus on, negative or positive. The saying "what you resist persists" couldn't be truer in regards to self-care: fight fat and fat will fight you right back.

Fitness is not a war, it's a relationship. How you take care of your whole self—your self-care (eating, exercise, health, feelings, state of mind, and spiritual connection)—is the most primary relationship in your life. From birth to death, it is with you. It is extremely significant—one of the most powerful relationships you'll ever know. You cannot keep pushing against, segregating, hating, avoiding, and abusing parts of yourself and expect to create a happy, easy, in-love-with-how-you-look relationship with your body. Love and long-term relationships don't work that way.

There is hope! Those without the mutated fitness chromosome can shift this whole dilemma by starting to think of self-care as a relationship or a marriage (or some other long-term, meaningful aspect of life, like parenting or career). Maybe your relationship is nonexistent or poorly managed, or could be it's on and off, or mean and abusive, or just blah—joyless. This relationship works the same as any important long-term commitment. It takes meaning, connection, presence, love, and willingness to make it work, and it has more to do with where you're at psycho-emotionally than anything else. It has ups and downs; occasionally there are things to be worked out or compromised upon. But this long-term relationship (LTR) with your body can be fantastic, simple, successful, and even easier than your "real" relationships.

Love Yourself Fit® is a different way to embark on this relationship with self. It's a guide to another path—the loving path. It's not another war book. There are no assigned eating programs or workout plans. It's a catalyst to a creating a healthy relationship with your body from the inside out. This book is a personal training manual for your mind. It will help you shift your perception, thoughts, feelings, and energy about your body, fitness, fat, exercise, and food. And it won't do it for you. If you want to shift to easy and enjoyable fitness, you have to take the baby steps to establish and cherish a love-based relationship each day.

If your self-care is a relationship you want to improve, then keep reading. The next three chapters clarify the divisive areas of your body relationship—the specific mindsets that ruin the relationship and maintain the war. The remainder of the book addresses each of these three areas and guides you to building a meaningful, enjoyable LTR with your body for life.

CHAPTER 2

Disconnection: The Cheating Mindset

"Where there's marriage without love,
there will be love without marriage."

Benjamin Franklin

Imagine you're sitting across the dinner table from the man you deeply love. You're married and committed to a lifetime together; you both want happily ever after. You cook and clean for him, take care of every aspect of your shared life, and do his bidding whatever it may be—tired, hungry, or sore you still show up. Your love knows no bounds. Tonight, like last night, he looks you in the eye and romantically proclaims his love and commitment to you and your relationship. He wants to love you fully and be the best partner you could possibly have.

Shortly after his enchanting speech, he gets up and opens the door for his lover. She sits down at the table with the two of you. Still babbling about wanting the best for the two of you, he caresses her leg and begins to kiss her. You would be shocked if this was a strange occurrence, but it isn't. It happens regularly, sometimes nightly. None the less, each time it happens you still feel violated. You quietly protest. You ask him nicely to stop; you tell him you don't want this. He doesn't listen. Unfortunately you have nowhere else to go, so as usual, you have to sit with his philandering until he's had his fill. As if his slobber fest with this home-wrecking tramp isn't enough, he stops kissing her long enough to say, "I'll be good to you tomorrow honey, promise."

Really? Does he really think this won't matter tomorrow? He's blatantly cheating on you! And he's asking you to sit there and be party to his indiscretions. In the midst of it all, he has the balls to claim he really cares about you; say he wants to be good to you and do what's best for you. What kind of asshole would do this and ask you to continue to put up with his philandering?

As the late night infomercial states, "But wait, there's more!"

Even more disturbing, his idea of being "good" to you is not loving or kind. Though he gives lip service to the opposite, your feelings, experiences, and the events of your life are irrelevant to him. To him the relationship is about him: his feelings, his desires, and his experiences. Unless you're interrupting or hurting him, he pretty much ignores you. He's not thinking long-term or of a mutually loving partnership (with you at least). He clearly takes you for granted. How could you stay with this asshole? In reality, you wouldn't. Even if he was the sexiest man on earth, loaded, and dynamite in bed you wouldn't stay with him.

Actually, you are him. The asshole adulterer is you. (Take a breath; I know—it's like trying to swallow a dry dog turd.) You and your body are in the identical relationship. You're treating your body the same way our imaginary adulterer treated you: without respect or love. You pretend that your actions and energy toward your body isn't impactful—as if there is no connection between your actions, thoughts, feelings, and body. You say you love your body and want to be good to it, and then you open the cupboard door for *your* lover (food) and start cheating by overeating!

Despite this disrespectful, unloving, and disconnected partnership, your body is stuck with you. It has no place else to go. You ignore your body's voice and indulge, thinking your indiscretions won't count tomorrow.

Your body is what a shrink would call codependent with you. It shows up for you every day, cooks, cleans, and does your bidding without complaint or often without a decent night's sleep. You ignore, take advantage, or outright abuse it daily, monthly, annually. Despite your actions, thoughts, or negative talk, your body shows up to grow hair, kill bacteria, create new cells, and all that other homeostatic stuff. Your body is there for you faithfully, because it only knows love, connection, and partnership (through function).

You are cheating on your body! (Slut!) You ignore your body's wellbeing, requests, and boundaries to indulge your psycho-emotional needs and cravings at your body's expense. Sexy food comes in the room and you're gone! As if a binge today doesn't count, you pause long enough to think or say, "Tomorrow I'll be good to you (body), promise." You wouldn't tolerate anyone else treating you this way, would you?

This disrespectful and disconnected approach is the first part of the collapse of your self-care. When it comes to self-care, separation between body, mind, and spirit manifests as failed undertakings and self-sabotage. There's a breakdown of integrity within you—one you can feel after you've heard the enchanting speech from your adulterer self a few times. Your intentions, desires, and actions clash and your body gets lost in the shuffle. It pays the price by way of a binge or a marathon. This separation makes everything about getting and staying in shape seem effortful, difficult, and forever inconsistent.

You are sabotaging yourself because your whole self is not on the same page. Just like the spouse who is unfaithful, you have an illusion of sep-arateness, but yours is between body and mind. You are in a disconnected state between thoughts, wants, feelings, sensations, and actions. This disconnection is exemplified when you know there's a better choice—one that aligns with your true intentions and your body's voice—but you choose otherwise. A healthy choice for dinner would be broccoli and lemon chicken, yet you opt for a bacon cheeseburger instead. A brisk walk would do your heart good, but you decide you deserve to watch TV. Your body is not hungry, but you eat twelve cookies because your heart is famished. You're not hungry, you're food horny! You're craving and eating out of boredom, wanting satisfaction, or avoiding something. You've gotten in the habit of self-indulgence when what you really want (or need) is self-nurturing or a deeper kind of nourishment.

If you have difficulty fitting in fitness, or you've been fighting to accomplish the same weight loss goal for months or years without lasting results, you're probably stuck in this type of energy draining, disconnected relationship. That's right, disconnection is energy draining. Being in a disconnected state scatters and consumes your energy. A disconnected, insane LTR takes a lot of energy. Haven't had one? Oh, they're a hoot. When you're dating someone crazy or live with a chaotic relationship, you'd better take your vitamins and eat your WHEATIES®, because the personal energy required to sustain a dysfunctional relationship is overwhelming. The insanity tends to ooze into other areas of your life too. Your work, other relationships, finances, and your self-esteem all seem more chaotic or demanding when you're involved with a whack job. No one can stay in a state of fighting and forcing for a lifetime and have a surplus of energy, time, resources, or really relax.

Not only is a disconnected, energy draining, and insane LTR horrible to live with, it also doesn't work. Big shocker! Be it sports, career, relationships, or personal goals, when disconnection and betrayal reign, chaos and failure soon follow. Have you ever heard of a football team winning the Super Bowl© with its players unorganized, not using the same play book, or running off to play for the other team? Of course not and that's a silly question, because you only watch the commercials. You won't ever hear of it happening, because "misaligned and disconnected" drains and devastates *anything it rules*—it doesn't work in any area of life. (Unless of course you're a branch of the federal government that can vote oneself a pay raise despite your inability to compromise or draw up a functioning budget. Apparently, chaos and insanity can work for certain entities.)

Congress aside, you're not alone in this misalignment. Many of us are so consumed with our daily lives that we're unaware of how disconnected we've become. In this era of rushed driving, instant meals, and crazy schedules, most of us have lost touch with our bodies. We don't listen to hunger or satiation cues; we eat when we're already full and starve when our stomachs rumble. We keep ourselves awake when we're tired and find it difficult to recall the joy we once found in running, playing, and moving our bodies. Today our choice of entertainment is seated, multisensory consumption. This imbalanced lifestyle creates a skewed scale, pulling us toward cycles of low energy, poor health, and a draw toward more consumption. We end up sabotaging ourselves in a lame attempt to nurture or reenergize ourselves by way of food, busyness, or plain avoidance.

Women in particular have a difficult time maintaining healthy space for self-care time. We seem to have developed the feminine legacy of submerging our own health and wellbeing beneath everyone and everything else in our lives. If you're like most, you probably spend more time running errands than you do improving your health or enjoying loved ones. Whether it's cleaning the cat box, driving the kids to soccer practice, or answering one of a thousand e-mails, body and spirit usually get neglected for things much less significant. You get so caught up in life's minutiae that you end up neglecting yourself and those elements of life that are most meaningful.

In the same vein, when hurt, uncomfortable, or anxious feelings arise you avoid them with overstimulation, distraction, or numbing out. How would you have learned otherwise? Did you have the Dealing with Feelings class in Jr. High School or get The "Brain Owner's Manual" for Christmas at age seven? Probably not. Your emotional etiquette was most likely absorbed from the family and society in which you grew up.

How is this relevant to your thighs? You're deciding what to feed them and how much to move them based on your psycho-emotional state. If you've never learned to acknowledge your psycho-emotional state, let alone deal with it, you won't be able to deal with food horny, your adulterer self, or the mean bitch in the bathroom mirror! You'll keep cheating on yourself and the war will continue, because a disconnected, misaligned, energy draining and insane mindset makes goals that are disconnected, misaligned, energy draining, and insane. Your inner living habits become your outer living habits.

Your body is not separate from your life or your mind. What's going on in your head, or schedule, or relationships is also happening in your body. There's a mountain of evidence in the discipline of Psychoneuroimmunology (PNI) supporting this mind-body connection in regards to health and disease. Study after study is piling up linking one's state of mind to one's state of health. If your state of mind can affect your immune function and heart health, consider the influence your mind-state may have on your metabolic rate or lipid utilization. I believe mind lives in the body as well as the brain therefore affects homeostasis and the everyday functions of the body, including weight. In time I believe we'll see more evidence emerge along these lines.

In our world today the era of separateness has passed on the micro and macro scales. The time has come to build a self-care practice based on a connected and aligned mind and body.

An aligned and sane LTR with your body will bridge your self-care divide by bringing your warring factions together for peace talks. This will be the focus of Sections II and III.

CHAPTER 3

Loveless Marriage: The Abusive Mindset

*"A great deal of intelligence can be invested in ignorance
when the need for illusion is deep."*

Saul Bellow

Imagine you had a dream about being in an abusive relationship. The man you're with is a prick and he treats you poorly, particularly in regards to your appearance. He constantly criticizes and berates you and you tolerate his obnoxious behavior. "Why can't you lose that disgusting fat?" he asks as he pinches the flesh of your waist. "This is gross," he sneers. As you get dressed for an evening out, he remarks, "I can't believe you're going to wear that—you look huge!" Yet, in the recent past he had forbid you from buying clothes that fit your body. "Lose some of that weight and you'll fit into your regular clothes," he says.

He's always commenting on the food you eat and nags you about going to the gym. Aloud he compares you to other women, yet sabotages you by bringing home cookies and ice cream for the two of you. When you go out, he only takes you to fast food places, as he claims he doesn't have enough time to take you anywhere "nice".

What if this was real life? How long would you tolerate his behavior? How would you feel being treated this way? I'm sure you have an image conjured up, or at least a few words you'd like to say to him at this point. But I'd like you to focus on his vibe or energy. What is it like being around him in your dream? Is your experience negative or positive? Did you get the loving, welcoming vibe or the bitter, averse feeling in his presence?

Wake up! He's you and you treat your body the same way the wanker in your dream treated you. Don't you constantly criticize yourself? Bitterly squeeze the fat rolls? Compare yourself to other women? Not allow time for a "nice" meal and then sabotage yourself with goodies? Restrict wardrobe additions until some measurement is satisfied? Don't forget all the conversations you have with your friends, or even strangers in public restrooms, about what an asshole your body has been, getting fat and old and all. Your energy and perspective are just as abusive as the loser in your dream.

Can you imagine a friend or your actual spouse treating you the way you treat your body with the demeaning comments, pinching, and comparisons? Or talking to strangers about how awful you look? How would that go over in your house? Not well I think! Imagine the way your body feels about all this poking, pinching, criticism, judgment, and sabotage every day from someone it can't get away from: you! Furthermore, if you were to start "taking care of yourself" from this mindset, your self-care practice wouldn't be a change of heart but pandering to the abuser within. Your ideas of being "good" to your body are on par with the bitter wanker: forceful, judgmental, and restrictive. As if you can nourish your body and mind with relentless dieting, counting, measuring, no carbs, no sugar, no-no-no, and only five ounces of wine, dear. Or perhaps you can nurture or energize yourself with a ridiculously exhausting exercise class with psycho-exer-Nazi lady. Chastise Class with the Suzi-Fitness app or evening assessments with the bitch in your bathroom mirror could lighten your heart and mind, but I doubt it. None of the above is good self-care.

The only way we have learned to "care" for our bodies is chastened.

You've developed a callous perspective and noxious relationship with your body over the course of your lifetime. This loveless marriage is a reflection of your mindset, culture, beliefs, and self-perception. According to John Gottman (big marriage guy in the psych world), doomed relationships display what he calls The Four Horsemen of the Apocalypse. Criticism, contempt, defensiveness, and stonewalling are the four characteristics displayed by ill-fated couples. Contempt, the biggest killer of love, includes name calling, obnoxious responses like eye rolling, and hostile or sarcastic humor. You may not treat your spouse this way, but don't you call your body names or say things like "fat-ass" or "flabby"? Perhaps you make faces, roll your eyes, or groan at your image in the mirror. Or occasionally make an unkind remark or joke at your body's expense. Congratulations! You have successfully seeded a garden of contempt toward your body and it's blossoming in your self-care relationship.

Being contemptuous or a "body abuser" in this society is not only accepted, it's practically encouraged. Women make a bonding ritual out of complaining about themselves. Bitching about fat thighs is a way to connect to other women. Women use body bitching to reassure other women. A good-looking woman will complain about her looks to assure other women of her perceived position in the herd—that she is not a threat. Another woman will complain—strictly for reassurance—that she is hideous or unlovable because of her appearance. Attractive or not, a negative body image is a way to keep each other feeling close and safe. It's part of our female subculture.

As a woman, the subject of beauty and one's body is a loaded one when uninvestigated. Female self-perception, value, esteem, and power are likened to one's appearance. A secret obsession with one's looks can be simultaneously controlling, intimidating, and embarrassing.

If you're very attractive, other women may feel intimidated and secretly wish you would ugly yourself up or pack on a few pounds so they might be more comfortable in your presence. (Oh, come on…admit it! You know at least one woman you wish would pack on thirty pounds or drool on herself while speaking to a group of people. Just once, God, please?) On the other hand, if a woman doesn't represent the ideal image of beauty, she's expected to take action to "fix" herself. If Suzy isn't good looking, she should lose weight, think about rhinoplasty, or color her hair. The unspoken rule of our society is that a woman should get as close to "perfect" as she can. It doesn't matter if she's a mother, teacher, doctor, or roofing contractor, that she's indifferent to social ideals, doesn't read magazines, or can't afford the luxury of pursuing beauty. She should try to look as beautiful as possible. In our world, a woman is programmed to believe that she's more acceptable, more successful, and more valuable if she's beautiful, young, or thin.

A large part of these beliefs and subsequent behaviors stem from popular culture. Pop culture, at current, doesn't value older, fatter, or "unattractive" people, particularly women. It may be hard to believe nowadays, but there were times when adults weren't made to look stupid in technology ads and female curves were thought to be attractive. To be considered "beautiful" or "attractive" today one must fit into the images narrowly defined by the culture. Older women, minorities, and more recently obese people complain about our country's lack of multi-dimensional images of beauty. Certainly not everyone has the same perception of who or what is beautiful. Yet most of us buy into the ideals and standards dictated to us without question.

Pop cultural ideals are born of an illusory world. This interconnected, media-infused world is alluring, titillating, and persuasive. Because the nature of media is so influential and pervasive (and because we're perpetually connected to a screen of some sort), we're constantly directed to the external aspects of our lives and of ourselves. The media, via the airbrush, Photoshop, or animation, has sold us a standard of "beauty" that's artificial and impossible, and therefore extremely destructive. I view this beauty standard as a tiny box, a "beauty box," into which temporarily fits about one tenth of one percent of us. This constant bombardment has come to influence our perspective, our choices, and what we value. We've become a society that values things and appearances over actual wellbeing or health.

This lack of substance in our cultural values is our own. It's not entirely the media's or the advertising industry's doing. We are the source. We keep the beauty box alive with every dollar we spend chasing beauty. You and I are the market; we're at least partly responsible for the social values and our feminine subculture. If we didn't fund the beauty box, it wouldn't exist!

Despite the irrational nature of our cultural mindset, you've probably invested a good part of your life struggling to squeeze yourself into this tiny box called *beautiful*. You spend time, money, and energy. If you fail, you turn to self-abuse, physically, psychologically, and emotionally. You become the abusive spouse, over or underdoing your self-care, instigating the loveless marriage. Your body then pays the price of cruel comments, negative emotions, and God-knows-what kinds of procedures, regimens, and diets.

This unloving relationship with the self begets a vicious cycle. Your perception turns your body into the enemy that must be punished into submission. You try to fix yourself by going to extremes like liquid diets, marathon workout sessions, or diet pills. The last thing you tried didn't work, so you think you have to try something else. There's a psycho-drama playing out in your mind, pushing you to the edge. Oh no, it's not…Oh yes it is: El Armario de Ropa Sucia! (The Closet of Dirty Clothes!) Your closet turns into a Latin soap opera every morning: crying, blame, cursing, smeared makeup, and sheer outrage. How dare those jeans feel so tight today when only last week they were so kind to your nalgas (buns), caressing them into a taunt-looking eighteen year-old form with no problema. Now you can't even get them over your hips! Chingar (F**k)!

The only way out of the closet Novela is to jump back on the pendulum and swing to the other extreme with the latest, craziest fitness fad.

This pendulous behavior pattern is underwritten by certain parts of the diet and fitness industries, not only by promoting trendy diets and selling get-fit-quick machines but in the use of beauty-box images as marketing and advertising tools. Diet and nutrition companies, equipment manufacturers, gyms, magazines, and various organizations and professionals promote these same images and take them to alarming extremes. A good part of the fitness industry—your would-be resource pool—is polluted with lookism.

As a consumer, you naively believe you can and should look like the fitness models on TV and in magazines if you would just exercise twenty minutes, three times a week on the magic machine. You believe it's reasonable to have ripped abs at age forty-seven by merely following the eleven easy steps on the back of the box. Or that you can lose weight and build muscle without exercising if you simply apply the pads to the area you want to slim down and turn on the machine; you'll watch as your muscles burn the fat away…Kool-Aid© anyone?

Many people, including professionals, believe one's physical appearance of fitness is paramount to actual fitness. However, most of the benefits of truly being fit are not obvious or visible like flexibility, strength, power, endurance, lower resting heart rate, lower blood pressure, heightened insulin sensitivity, and most importantly, feeling good. Those infected with lookism are convinced that "looking fit" is the same as "being fit." Some of the fittest *looking* people are using imbalanced eating, drugs, starving, steroids, overtraining, or dealing with a plethora of injuries to look fit. In truth, beauty-box images don't help you get fit, they only contribute to pendulous behavior swings, establish an air of perfectionism, and increase negative feelings and self-talk. Put down the fruit drink and walk away!

Besides, super fit looking people can be fairly obsessive about their bodies, hateful of fat, and quite controlling about what they eat. They often teach the same principles: obsess, hate, and control. So even if you lose weight or meet your goals under these principles, you must obsess, hate, and control yourself into staying that way. If war is how you got there, war is how you stay.

While good health remains secondary to beauty, many people will find themselves stuck in a painful cycle of on-and-off programs that never deliver permanent results. The beauty box is externally conceived and therefore an extrinsic motivator for most people. It's a well-known fact among health behavior experts that *extrinsic motivation lacks longevity and power*. External remediation does not remedy the source of your problem: perceptual distortions, emotional interference, and negative behavior patterns. Rather it acts as the Band-Aid® for the carcinoma—covering but not healing. On-and-off fitness feeds the loveless marriage, creates more self-flagellation, and leads to more failing cycles.

A loveless marriage is a miserable way to live. You can't hate, beat, or abuse someone into an effortless, loving relationship. You can't hate, beat, or abuse your body into being pretty enough for you to love it. Like an abusive spouse, this type of relationship with your body is painful to live with and only becomes increasingly destructive with time. Therefore, one of the most important components to creating easy, flowing self-care is love. Genuine respect or love for your body makes self-care effortless.

In Section IV, Building a Loving Relationship Together, we'll dive into creating a loving relationship.

CHAPTER 4

Arrival Thinking:
The Get-the-Ring Mindset

"It is a woman's business to get married as soon as possible, and a man's to keep unmarried as long as possible."

George Bernard Shaw

Remember when you met that special someone and he sent a chill down your spine and a flutter through your heart? Meeting him, you felt the most basic and primal of feelings: lust. Relationships often start with this phase of wild passion, during which one's anticipation and emotions are at their height.

You jump into this would-be relationship visualizing love blossoming into happily ever after. You start picking out your flowers and his tux. This frenzy of feelings and hormones inspires you to do things at a pace you normally would not. You stay up all night talking or making love when you're due at the office at 8 a.m. Although you can't afford it, you give him an expensive watch for Valentine's Day. You dress up in something sexy and make him a gourmet dinner. Whatever you do in this honeymoon phase, it's most probably not how you would behave in a long-term relationship.

A new romance is a good example of what I call the emotional jump start.

The emotional jump start is motivation based on the excitement and passion you're experiencing; it's emotion that literally jump starts you. It's not the reality of a lifelong relationship but the fairytale fantasy of romance and happily ever after. It's lusty and urgent, want-it-all-now with disregard for living in reality. In a realistic relationship, he may pee on the toilet seat and fart in his sleep. She may be a terrible cook and wear grandma panties. In a real LTR there will be joyful moments and shared triumphs, but there will also be issues, arguments, and tougher times. An LTR is considerate and patient and functions well in the embrace of reality.

The emotional jump start—the passion you feel so strongly in the beginning—won't keep you committed when everyday reality sets in. A late bill, grumpy morning, or any number of in-law issues can dry things right up! You may be dreaming about your wedding day, but you'll need more than lusty emotion to make the marriage last. The dynamics that foster a person's willingness to stay with a relationship through its inevitable ups and downs isn't lust, romance, or expensive gifts. It's deeper than that. A lasting LTR has depth, meaning, satisfaction, love, joy, partnership, and much more.

For many of us fitness has the same emotional jump start as a new romance. First comes the meeting of an idea: molding oneself into the perfect physical specimen. The excitement phase includes a fantasy or two about the attention you'll get, or the confidence you'll feel with your dynamite new body. "I'm gonna be skinny, bitches!" you shout with your inside voice as you eagerly introduce your new diet to girlfriends. You eagerly anticipate the admiration and pride that will accompany your new physique as you daydream about turning heads in pants so tight you can only jam yourself into them with motor oil. Spandex and sequins baby! (Not that you would, but in your aggrandizing weight loss hallucinations, you could.) You dream about taking clothes shopping to the abusive level.

You chuckle aloud as you envision an orgy for your credit card: a series of nameless, faceless encounters with swipe machines as you stock your closet with new, tight fitting, skinny-girl clothes.

With all this passion and energy churning inside, you jump into doing things you normally would think are crazy. You might put yourself on the grapefruit-and-bacon diet, sign up for a 5:30 a.m. kickboxing class, or spend forty dollars on gluten-soy-sugar-dairy-free crackers. Whichever you choose, it's probably not how you would spend your energy, time, money, or stomach space long-term. With the fantasy of your perfect body driving you, you convince yourself your new plan is going to work no matter how impractical or miserable the daily practice may be. Because he—I mean this diet — is the one!

Like any relationship based on the superficial, your fitness lust usually dies when everyday reality kicks in. It may last three days or three weeks, but the severe get-fit-quick program usually doesn't survive more than a couple of months. You've probably experienced the fallout of the emotional jump start. The downfall begins with missing the 5:30 a.m. aerobics class, so you guilt yourself into going to the gym after work. Cursing the step machine with each step you take, you leave feeling irritable, tired, and thanking God it's over. By the time you get home you're starving, and you scour the cupboards for something to eat—anything to eat but grapefruit and bacon! You find something like the kids' snack packs or settle for tubes of cheese spread on the forty dollar cardboard you bought, and you stuff yourself. You fall into bed feeling frustrated and thoroughly disgusted with yourself, promising to start anew in the morning ...or maybe Monday...or perhaps next week...or...

The original lust or emotional jump start won't keep you committed when everyday reality kicks in. You want happily-ever-healthy—a marriage, not a one-night stand! You're looking for long-term! Grapefruit and bacon won't cut it as everyday cuisine, and you better be a perky morning person to skip coffee and be at kickboxing by 5:30 a.m. every day. And the forty dollar everything-free crackers speak for themselves. Urgency and get-the-ring thinking doesn't work for long-term partnerships.

The emotional jump start and subsequent fallout is from what I call arrival thinking. Whether it's a romantic relationship or your personal fitness plan, when you start with only the destination in mind, the journey gets neglected. "Getting-the-ring" doesn't make a relationship lovely or permanent, and your fixation on it would definitely screw up a first date and the entire relationship. Wedding day or goal weight, when the arrival is all that matters then the arrival takes precedence over the actual relationship with your mate or the way you treat your body. You become so consumed with the outcome, you forget that you've integrated a living hell into your everyday life—or his.

Arrival thinking is deadly to fitness resolutions, because fitness is *not a destination*. Fitness is a constant state of being. "Being fit" comes with issues, joyful moments, stalemates, triumphs, boring days, and tougher times—just like a relationship. The reality of your life, and therefore your ongoing self-care, will include vacations, holidays, hormone-Olympics, and one word: Brie. Therefore you must create a fitness program that's everyday-oriented and grounded in what will work for you long-term. Just like your ideal mate, you've got to be able to live with him or it every day! You need more than a fantasy destination or an emotional oomph to keep you committed.

You can still set goals. Setting goals or intentions is different from arrival thinking. A goal becomes arrival thinking when you're so attached to the outcome that you're neglectful of yourself or others in the process. Wanting and planning a fabulous wedding is a marvelous thing. The problem arises when the bride is so mentally affixed to a specific outcome that she forgets the wedding is a celebration of a relationship with another person (who's probably in the room, listening to a lot of yelling about the florist being an incompetent asshole). In other words, if you're plan-ning a one hundred twenty thousand dollar wedding for an unstable or superficial relationship—confusing a fabulous wedding with a fabulous marriage—or become a Bridezilla because your flowers are the wrong shade of periwinkle, you're neglecting the living part of the experience. You're condemning yourself—and likely your spouse—to a painful process. The same is true for fitness. If you're spending five thousand dollars on a personal trainer and food program—confusing a fabulous number on the scale with living a healthy and fit life you enjoy—or you're obsessed with some numerical measurement of your body, you're neglecting the reality of your experience. You're condemning yourself, and your body, to a miserable process.

Actually, arrival thinking can be useful for some situations in life, but not for long-term self-care. Marathons yes, new eating plan no. Final exams yes, everyday workout no. Weeding the yard yes, facing the bitch in the mirror no. If you try to use arrival thinking for long-term situations, you'll end up feeling frustrated, deprived, and eventually you'll rebel. You won't fall, you'll jump off the wagon.

Attachment to outcome, urgency, and resistance to the present typify arrival thinking, but they're merely a mindset. Arrival thinking is an energy and state of mind, and it's your perspective that determines your experience on the path you walk.

Fitness, like a marriage, a career, or parenthood, is a lifelong endeavor and thrives when it's handled as such. A relationship doesn't consist of the day you meet someone and the day you break up. It's every day in between that's the relationship. Giving birth doesn't make you a parent; being a parent means making decisions, taking actions, and practicing certain behaviors you'll do the rest of your life. Getting a job doesn't earn you a career. A career only begins the day you start working. And an effective fitness course has no "first day" and "reach-your-goal-weight day"; there's only every day. Life isn't about arriving at a destination, and neither is fitness. You can't fall off the wagon if you're skipping alongside it, picking flowers. That's the focus of Section V, Healthy Ever After: The Practice.

SECTION II

Rekindling Connection & Learning How to Communicate

CHAPTER 5

Understanding Connections: Mind-Body Foundation

*"Some circumstantial evidence is very strong,
as when you find a trout in the milk."*

Henry David Thoreau

Recognizing the connections within you and your life environment is the foundation of building a relationship that will allow you to successfully bridge the great divide and rekindle the connection with your body. The next few chapters ask you to examine the link between your thoughts, feelings, and all of your life and offers tools to better affect the totality of your self-care.

Tangible Connections

In humans, everything is connected. Organs don't work independently of one another, and systems can't function void of each other. Nothing in your body, person, or lifestyle operates independently of the others. Your daily life affects your thoughts and feelings. Thoughts and feelings can create stress. Stress impacts digestion, heart rhythm, and immune function.

It's not a foreign concept that humans are thoroughly inner- and interconnected. When it comes to the mind and spirit, however, failure to recognize the connections has delayed the evolution of Western thought. The tangible, physical world belongs to science, and the intangible world belongs to the realm of religion or hocus pocus. Until recently, much of science has been focused on finding tangible results in physical bodies. Scientists haven't had the desire or tools to identify the "intangible" components that affect human health, like emotions and thoughts. Since the invention of the scientific method, the mind-body-spirit connection has been considered the unfounded babble of crystal wearers and solstice worshipers. Fortunately, Western mind-body research has been growing in popularity over the last thirty years and, with building evidence, is becoming more accepted by the mainstream medical and scientific communities.

Immune dysfunction, heart disease, digestive disorders, and diabetes are just a few of the top afflictions from which many suffer, and all are affected by not just one's physical health and course of treatment, but also by one's mental, emotional, and (possibly) spiritual state. In the fifties, Hans Selye proved that chronic stress can cause adrenal and immune dysfunction. In the seventies, Robert Adler conditioned rats to physiologically lower their immune response via an external stimulus. In the eighties, David Spiegel found that group therapy prolonged the lives of women with terminal breast cancer. These are a few examples of foundational milestones in mind-body research that have paved the way for further study and preventative medical measures. Research in the area continues to thrive, with a mountain of evidence driving it. In other words, the separation previously made between psychology and physiology is dissipating, even in some of the staunchest of medical arenas.

The work of the many practitioners and scientists who have promoted a theory of mind-body-spirit connection like Norman Cousins, Herbert Benson, Louise Hay, Andrew Weil, Candace Pert, Deepak Chopra, and Christiane Northrup has contributed to the development of the mind-body health model. Meanwhile, thousands of researchers and physicians are currently digging even deeper into the molecular connections and biochemistry between mind-state and physical health, and they're reaching amazing conclusions. As introduced in Chapter 2, this blossoming field is called Psychoneuroimmunology (PNI). PNI is producing eye-opening results about the way human emotion and thought directly impact physiology and affect the way we practice medicine.

For example, the traditional medical model has been that the brain is the supreme commander of communications within the body, reigning independent of thought or emotion. However, the research of Dr. Candice Pert and countless others has shown that information flows in all directions simultaneously, not merely from the brain to a muscle. Thus, the mind doesn't reside in the brain alone, but in the entire body. Moreover, the communication is directed by many influences, including one's psycho-emotional state. We could now claim that the body (physiology), heart (emotions), and brain (thought) together comprise the "mind".

If the mind doesn't dominate the body, nor the body dominate the mind, then we'll consider them partners: the mind and body are married as one being—you! This mind-body oneness is significant to those of us seeking to make physiological changes, because it means that our thoughts and feelings are as much in our bodies as they are in our heads or hearts. Your anger, sadness, or joy is traveling around with the blood cells in your body, influencing and directing the path and life of these cells. The stress related to your work is impacting the rhythm of your heart, your blood pressure, and the supply of oxygen your muscles receive. Conversely, the amount of laughter and joy in your life can boost your immune function, reduce inflammation, and lengthen your life span.

If psycho-emotional state so dramatically affects health and immunity, then how might it impact fitness? Does sadness, joy, or negative self-regard affect your ability to perform a challenging physical task? Could your mood change the way you digest your food or utilize fat for energy? Can different mind-states yield different postural deviations?

An interesting place to begin answering these questions relates to a more recent subject of PNI research on the body's inflammatory response. There's mounting evidence that negative emotions such as anxiety and depression contribute to immune system deregulation through the production of inflammatory substances called cytokines. Pro-inflammatory cytokines are believed to play a role in numerous chronic diseases, in general physical decline as we age, and may also interfere with healing musculoskeletal injuries, as these cytokines are suspect in contributing to muscle atrophy and hindering muscle repair.[1,2,3,4]

If state of mind can facilitate or disable disease and impact the musculo-skeletal system, then it's reasonable to consider that one's mind-state could influence one's fitness and wellbeing. Could your thoughts and feelings actually be affecting your physique? Could worrying regularly decrease your body's ability to build or maintain muscle? What if criticizing your physique is contributing to your body's fat-hoarding composition? Yes, I'm suggesting that your brain is attached to your body by way of this unique body part we'll call the neck. This amazing "neck" allows thoughts and emotions, possibly in the form of peptides and neurotransmitters, to communicate with the rest of the body. It's a strange concept, I know, but being a bitch to yourself could actually affect your physiology.

As of this writing, we don't yet know the answers to all these questions. But science may be answering affirmatively. For example, you may be familiar with the connection between cortisol and body fat. Cortisol is a hormone that your body produces when you experience psycho-emotional stress. Higher levels of cortisol hinder your body in using fat.[5] As you lower your stress levels, your levels of cortisol drop, allowing your body to access and utilize stored fat more readily. Hypothetically then, the less stress you experience, the less superfluous flesh you'll have around your middle. Yay relaxation!

There's an overwhelming amount of evidence that demonstrates a link between mind-state and body health, and I believe there's much more to come. With mind-state affecting disease and wellness as dramatically as research indicates, those of us attempting to improve health and body composition can't ignore this evidence in our pursuit of fitness. The dawn is breaking on the illusion of mind-body separateness, and the connection is becoming clearer.

Understanding Unseen Connections

Haven't you snapped at your mate out of stress or aggravation even though your mood had little to do with him? Maybe you've barked at the kids for some menial mistake. Or, far-fetched as it may be, perhaps you've been less than hospitable to a telephone solicitor once or twice. Whichever the case, your life is difficult to segment into separate categories and keep each part segregated from one another, or your state of mind.

Your self-care choices relate directly to what's going on inside of you and in your life. Mind, body, spirit, and lifestyle (MBSL) are all connected and all affect each other. Just like a relationship, these connections determine your everyday choices and therefore your outcome.

We know the body affects the mind. Exercising releases endorphins, and endorphins cause an elevation in mood. Flying can dehydrate the body, which in turn affects your brain's decision-making abilities and contributes to jet lag. Many studies have shown the detrimental effects of sleep deprivation or rotating-shift work on problem-solving abilities. The physiological mechanisms behind what used to be thought of as purely psychological, emotional, or spiritual disorders such as depression and schizophrenia are now effectively treated with medication and exercise.

Physiology affects psycho-emotional wellbeing and vice versa.

We now know the mind affects the body. One of the oldest and best examples is the placebo effect. Countless studies have shown that a person who takes a placebo can experience the same physiological changes as a person who takes a real drug. The patient believes the pill he has taken is medication, and his body responds by alleviating or diminishing the symptoms of his ailment. (Pharmaceutical companies love placebo effect! Actually my understanding is that they have a loathe-hate relationship with placebo, because it—the power of your mind—gets in the way of determining if you can be healed without *you* getting involved. Ah, the irony.)

Another example of the mind's power relates to the "fight-or-flight" response of the peripheral nervous system. Just the thought of danger can cause measurable physiological reactions, including the instantaneous release of adrenaline, elevation in heart rate, and even an epidermal reaction. Don't believe it? Think back to the last time you watched a scary movie—remember your heart racing and palms sweating? Truth to the mind becomes reality in the body.

You may have had a personal experience regarding a lifestyle choice affecting your feelings and mind-state. For example, if one of your goals is weight loss, when you overeat or blow off exercise you feel guilty. Conversely, if you choose to eat a healthy, light dinner and do the forty-minute workout you've committed to, you'll go to bed feeling good and awaken inspired the next day. Simply telling yourself a story about your actions—good or bad—moves you in one direction or the other. Your psycho-emotional wellbeing dramatically affects the choices you make, and the decisions you make influence the way you feel.

Another influence is that of environment. Have you ever noticed that when your kitchen or office is a mess you feel out of sync? Does the dent in your car door make you feel tired or frustrated every time you see it?

Maybe you've had to deal with a strained work environment, and you find yourself dreading going to the office. There's a unique connection between a person's surroundings and state of mind. An undefined correlation exists between peace of mind and environmental chaos, clutter, tension, damaged goods, and incomplete projects; these are just a few of the minute lifestyle annoyances that can affect one's mind-state. Likewise, the same is true in reverse: a tense, annoyed, or cluttered mind can create environments or a lifestyle in its likeness.

So what does all this mind-body connection mumbo-jumbo have to do with your waistline? You need to understand where your know-do disconnect is originating. Until now you've been thinking the solution is out there: you don't have the right diet, or workout, or shoes. However, if you have a goal, know what's required to meet that goal, and struggle for years or decades to maintain those requirements—in this case behaviors—then the problem isn't coming from anything outside of you. As if you were a computer running a virus in the background of your mind, the knowing isn't reaching the doing, because there are parts of you running interference on your unexamined MBSL connections.

An excellent example of the multidirectional connections of one's MBSL is eating. Prompts to eat can come from the body (physiological), the mind (thoughts or feelings), and lifestyle or environmental influences (time to eat lunch, holidays, "that lasagna smells good," or just sitting with food in front of you, picture Chris Farley on SNL: "Back off, I'm starving!"). Conversely, what you eat can affect the physiological mechanisms that act on brain function, mood, and sleep quality. Physiological hunger, felt strongly enough, can induce extreme behavior, while for most, emotions play a role in determining what, when, and how much one eats.

The connections between MBSL are multidirectional and easy to see when you look for them. Each simultaneously influences the other, resulting in your food choices and exercise behaviors. Recognizing the effects of the mind-body-spirit-environment on your fitness is the first step to rekindling your body connection and creating lasting fitness.

Your first workout begins now! This ⌘ means it's exercise time. You will use these exercises to put together your self-care practice, so save a digital or hard copy.

⌘ **Mental Fitness Exercise:** Write out how you feel about your body, exercise, and food as if they were people. Describe your relationship, how you get along, and what your opinion of them is. Thoughts, feelings, and beliefs are all good. Describe your energy or vibes about this area.

⌘ **Mental Fitness Exercise:** Write down what you would like that relationship to be on a daily basis. How would you feel? What would you like to think and believe? How would you behave?

⌘ **Mental Fitness Exercise:** How will you know when you're at peace with your body, exercise, and food? Describe your self-care as if it were a relationship; describe specifically how you want to feel in this relationship. Focus on your experience; forget numbers and the how-to-get-there strategy.

Go to www.loveyourselffit.com/inspiration for a downloadable version of these exercises.

CHAPTER 6

Feminine Philandering: Identifying Your Inner Saboteur

*"Boundaries aren't all bad. That's why there are
walls around mental institutions."*

Peggy Noonan

Now that you're aware of the connectedness of your MBSL, you can begin to investigate how these multidirectional connections affect *your* personal self-care.

Most fitness programs focus solely on the superficial aspects of one's lifestyle. Traditionally they delve deeply into how to change your physical environments to manipulate you into different behaviors: throw out all your junk food, hang a size 3 bikini on the fridge, and join an overpriced gym. This environmental manipulation isn't a bad thing; in fact it's very helpful to create a supportive environment. But it's not the whole picture—not enough to keep you from buying more junk food or roasting marshmallows over that size 3 bikini after you light it on fire. Your environments constantly change, and most of the time you have little control over your surroundings—in terms of goodies brought into your office, food commercials and billboards, appetizers at a party, aromas when you walk thru a mall, etc. In any environment you only have control over yourself. It makes sense then to focus on you—your mental environment—not your physical environment.

To begin addressing your mental environment, you'll identify the connections in your life that are affecting your choices. I like to think of this as running a virus scan on your computer. When your computer isn't executing your requests, you know there's something going on with it. It's likely a virus. Should you be afraid to run a scan or take it in for service? Does it mean your computer is screwed or trash? Of course not. Your computer is fine; it simply needs the sabotaging programming removed. To do so, you have to identify which programs are causing problems.

If you have struggled with the know-do part of fitness, food, and weight, there's more going into your choices and self-sabotage than the boxes in your pantry. You need a scan of your mindset. Should you be afraid of your thoughts and feelings? Does it mean you are screwed or trash if you have sabotaging programming running in the background? Of course not. You're fine honey; you simply need to identify your thought viruses and clean up your programming.

Philandering and Boundaries

How many times have you asked yourself, "What's my problem? I'm smart, reasonably successful, and able to maintain other parts of my life—why not this exercise and eating thing?"

This fitness-eating-weight loss-self-care relationship is wholly connected and interdependent with the inner you. While your body is in a committed and monogamous LTR, you've mostly given this marriage lip service and run your self-care as if it were a cursory, open marriage. As you probably know, relationships like this don't work. A healthy relationship has agreements and boundaries *both* parties honor. As a part of a satisfying coupling, you can mend that which is out of alignment with your shared highest good and best self-care. In so doing, you make the choice to become conscious of those places where you may unconsciously hold yourself back or sabotage yourself.

The majority of us ladies haven't learned to establish healthy boundaries in mind, body, or lifestyle. Our thoughts, schedules, relationships, and belongings overwhelm us regularly. Terminally hungry for more, we continue to stuff our lives with "yeses" to things, people, and consumables. We can't manage the belongings we have, but we buy more. Without paying off our credit cards, we head to the malls for more shopping. We're challenged by the weight around our middles, yet we indulge daily. (The exception to all of this, of course, is when you do see the perfect pair of boots, and then all this philosophical stuff flies, not walks, out the window. And you have my full support on that occasion!)

In reality, this imbalanced perspective directs our energy, priorities, and relationship to self. The average American woman today has extremely high expectations for herself. She should be a great friend, daughter, and/ or sister. She also thinks she should be a perfect mother, an ideal wife, and a stunning beauty with a Barbie-perfect body. Her accomplishments shouldn't end there however; she needs to be a success in the boardroom, bedroom, and kitchen, and must have made her mark as a philanthropist. She needs to keep up on current events, hip blogs, and be a fashion maven. And if she wants to be cool, she should be doing yoga, HIIT, or Pilates. All of the above must be maintained with a keenly balanced mental-emotional state and an essence of goodwill towards all mankind, without anger, prejudice, or body fat.

Seriously? We expect too much from ourselves and naively believe that we can be, do, and have all of the above, every day. We're perfectionists. Ironically, we tend to put ourselves last on the priority list. How can one expect herself to be everything from philanthropic role model to Pilates sex goddess, while she remains the lowest one on the totem pole? How can we do it? We can't! Still, we try, and leave in our wake less than healthy bodies, mental and emotional ill-being, and spiritual disconnection.

Many of my female clients have a huge problem making fitness a permanent part of their lives, because they don't give themselves self-care time. Everyone and everything gets scheduled in their itinerary before the smallest effort toward self-nurturing. A workout, a bubble bath, a good book, meditation, toenails, and sometimes even a hot, seated meal are on permanent hiatus. "I don't have time!" is the too-common mantra of today's woman. I once had a client tell me that she would go home at night with an aching bladder because she wouldn't take the time to urinate her entire workday. But who's in charge of your daily allotment of time? Your husband, children, boss, or mother? Your husband, mother, and kids aren't shoveling brownies down your throat or asking you to relinquish a ten-minute walk during your lunch hour. Neither is your boss. If you have time to watch television, read, or post photos and online updates for more than ten minutes a day, then "I don't have time for self-care" is bullshit. Most of your life has been automated, and you've chosen to fill your time with other things. You may be strapped for time in your full life, but "I don't *want* to make time for this myself" is a more appropriate answer. No one is making your schedule but you, and sister, it's time you're honest with yourself about this.

For many of us overscheduling or overdoing has become an addiction. Like booze to the alcoholic, we continue to give our lives away in small increments, seeking a dose of feel-good with each commitment. Then we tend to be dishonest with ourselves about it, as if the world around us requires us to be up until 12:30 a.m. making cookies for the morning PTA event. This seemingly female-specific disease, which I call feminine philandering, leaves many of us overwhelmed, depressed, anxious, stressed out, attention-deprived, needy, and physically unhealthy. Like an unfaithful spouse, we betray ourselves.

How many times have you used food as a break, energy supplement, or reward instead of a nap, a walk, or healthy self-nurturing? How often have you blown off the gym because you felt too exhausted or fed up to go? How often have you found yourself frustrated in a nonessential commitment you made to another person or organization? Be honest. Without the willingness to say "no" and allow clear space for your self-care, you'll continue to struggle, war, and philander.

Like most addictions, feminine philandering for you may have become not only a coping mechanism, but a way to remain detached about the state of your life. If you continue to stay busy with everything and everyone around you, you'll never have to look at yourself—the source of the feelings, choices, behaviors, and lifestyle you're maintaining. This is one of those viruses running on your mental hard drive which keeps your self-care blocks hidden and the disconnect intact.

Boundaries: Making Space for You

How do you stop your cheatin' heart? The solution to feminine philandering is creating a clear space for you to operate—boundaries, in other words. Establishing boundaries is simply saying no gracefully to the things that conflict with your highest good. It doesn't have to be an all-out war or grueling climb up the Himalayas. Being true to yourself is for your highest good (and your children's, spouse's, company's, etc.). It's the foundation of true self-care.

You can't develop a relationship with another person unless you make time to spend together. You won't be able to grow your relationship with your body unless you allow time for it. I can't count the number of times I've heard a philandering new client say, "I just need to get into the habit of exercising." In reality, the first habit for this person to develop is not daily exercise or disciplined eating but the habit of allowing space for herself and being true to herself.

To begin the be-true-to-you process, the first thing you'll want to do is banish Superwoman from your perceptive reality. She doesn't exist. If you see a woman wearing what looks to be a cape, it's not. It's a really ugly, oversized scarf. Somewhere, sometime, something has to give. It may be health, psychological wellbeing, relationships, or the kids—but something has to get put on the back burner.

A great example of feminine philandering, a.k.a. holding on to Super-woman, is my own experience with becoming a mother. I had always fancied myself a career woman—independent and industrious. When I got pregnant, I got scared. I thought I would lose my career and my freedom. I didn't know how I was going to get it all done: maintain my business, marriage, and home; finish this book; and care for an infant. Shortly after giving birth, I was feeling stressed. Even though it was financially more prudent for me to stay home than to pay for infant care, I was afraid. Discussing my fears with my mother, I attempted to verbally strategize a return to work.

"Honey," she said, "your daughter will only be four months old once in your lifetime. She will only take a step, use a spoon, and smile for the first time once! You can't get back this first year, ever." She wisely continued, "Your career will always be available and waiting for your return. It's not going anywhere. And you don't realize this now, but this year will fly by, and before you know it Gillian will be off to school, and you'll be wishing you had taken all the time you could have with her when she was little."

I knew in my gut she was right. And I knew there was more to my eagerness and angst. I realized that I was trying to rush back to work out of fear. I was afraid of losing ground, letting go of my independence and income. Like so many women today, I wanted to do it all, because I thought I would miss out on something if I didn't. My actions were not coming from my values and spirit, but from fear that I would be less than, fall behind, or miss something if I "limited myself" to mom and wife.

I was able to let go of trying to do it all right now with an infant. I still remind myself that my peace is more important; my kids, marriage, and self-care are all more important. I can do it all…in time. I can't do and have it all at the same time, unless I'm willing to sacrifice the quality of some aspect of my life. Shifting is a process. One piece at a time I started saying no to my career eight years ago, and now, one piece at a time, I'm doing it with other areas of my life that are overwhelming or fear driven.

Decide if your everyday experience—how you think and feel—is more valuable than the concept of perfection. Your daily experience and well-being, or content of your life, is more valuable than your to-do list, the laundry, weeding the yard, posting online, or fulfilling extemporaneous requests from the dog park association. The best way to get started on this is to ask yourself if the item in front of you is a love-based choice or a fear-based choice. Where is your "yes" coming from: spirit or ego? Love or fear? Untie the ugly scarf from your neck and become selective about what you spend your mind, time, and life on. Because right now, Superwoman is only a hero to your ego.

Just say "no"! You have the self-preservative right to say no to things that impinge on your health and wellbeing. Assign your self-care a specific time in your digital or personal organizer, and make it as important as a professional meeting or family obligation. Treat it as a date. Schedule it on paper or screen (and you'll be lean, if you know what I mean). Make it clear to others that you have another commitment at that time. I heard Dr. Christiane Northrup in a lecture once say, "Just say, 'I simply can't.'" "I have an appointment at that time" works well for me. Breaking appointments with yourself doesn't contribute to your self-esteem, goals or career, or make you a better caretaker. You're just as important as the dry cleaning, the dog's trip to the vet, and soccer practice.

Think about how you would feel if the guy you were interested in kept cancelling dates with you. Hurt? Disappointed? Angry? Insecure about the relationship? You wouldn't believe him if he said, "I swear I care about you. I am interested. Let's meet tomorrow," followed by another no-show. His continued lip service cancelation policy would eventually cause you to lose faith and walk away. Consider how your body feels after years of similar self-care stand-ups. If there's no trust in word and deed, there's no relationship. How can you have a good thing if one of you won't even show up?

Self-care stand-ups send the message to your body, the universe, and the people in your life: *I'm not important enough or worth showing up for.* You teach people how they can treat you (and your body) by the way *you* treat you.

Certainly you'll have obligations and responsibilities that you can't ignore to go to spin class or to make a tofu salad. However, you can effectively incorporate your self-care into your life today in small increments. This is the second step in rekindling your relationship with your body: make time for your "dates" together.

There are thousands of ways to use your life and responsibilities to support your self-care space. The more restrictive your schedule, the more creative you'll need to be. In my house we sometimes have a family dance party on Friday nights. We crank up the iPod and dance for twenty minutes or two hours. It's a blast! Think creatively about how you could incorporate movement with the whole family or friends. Take the family for a walk after dinner. Dance around the living room before work, or do lunges while you vacuum. Put a stationary bike in front of the TV and ride it while watching a program or the news. If you're stuck, get help.

Ask your kids or mate to help you devise a self-care plan, and they'll be more likely to respect it.

Think baby steps: add just ten minutes of meditation or walking, one serving of green veggies, or three deep breaths in the morning. Add one more per day or week. Before you know it, you'll be in full self-care practice and feeling the benefits thereof. Don't make it complicated; make it simple. Obsessing about reducing is as ridiculous as overindulging. Create space for yourself ten minutes at a time. Self-care, like a mate, shouldn't move into your house on the first date or be painful to fit into your life. It should become gradually more appealing with small doses and feel like a good match for your whole self.

To move forward on identifying your blocks to great self-care, you must identify exactly which areas of your life lack boundaries or need your attention.

The Life Wheel a.k.a. Virus Scan!

You know sex is all in your head, right? It takes more than rubbing tingly places to get most women off. Therefore, if you're having a difficult time enjoying sex, you probably understand that the source of said difficulties is not likely physical. Usually there are blocks within the mind or relationship that are manifesting in the bedroom. The place to begin seeking a solution then is not in bed, but on the couch! Likewise, when it comes to maintaining self-care, the problem is rarely physical. There are often blocks within you that are manifesting in your exercise and eating habits. Therefore, it's wise not to seek solutions in the gym, but rather on the proverbial couch—within yourself.

Draw a two-inch circle in the middle of a piece of paper. Draw seven rays emanating from the circle. Now label the rays as follows: *body (physical)*, *mind (or psycho-emotional wellbeing), career/contribution, relationships (all of them), finances, spirit, and environments.* You'll be marking your perceptions of or feelings about each area of your life. When you're finished it will look like a good, old-fashioned wagon wheel. Think of the base of the ray (nearest the circle) as having the most negative feelings or being the lowest rating and the tip of the ray as the areas you're most happy with or highest rating. Rate where you feel you're at with each of these areas by placing a dot on each ray.

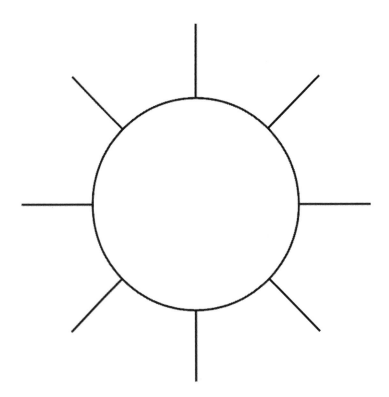

Each dot would include the obvious elements of that area of your life as well as your thoughts and feelings about said part of your life or self. The body, for instance, would include your current physical condition, self-care program or habits, and your thoughts and feelings about your body. When determining a spoke's rating, you could ask yourself questions like: Is my career/work a positive place to spend my time? Am I using my innate talents? Are my relationships honest and enjoyable or am I dreading the holidays with my family? Is there an unfinished project begging to be completed? Get the idea? Once you've marked each ray, connect the dots, each to the one next to it until you have a second circle, sort of.

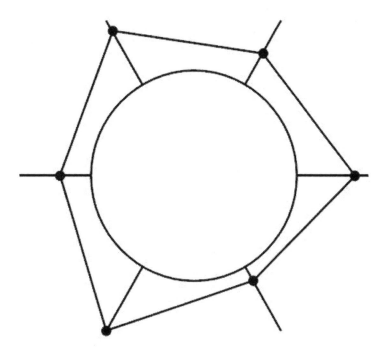

You've drawn a wheel representative of your life—like a wagon wheel with each ray being a life spoke. Consider this wheel a real one. Could you drive on it? Probably not! Each short life spoke creates a rougher ride and puts more stress on the other spokes and on the wheel as a whole. When your wheel is unbalanced or lopsided your forward motion is impeded, momentum is lost, and your engine energy is drained.

At first glance, it might seem as if your life spokes are independent of each other. But if you think about each of these spokes in relation to your everyday life, you'll understand how each affects the other. If you're experiencing an upset in your primary relationship, it will show in your performance at work and in your emotional wellbeing. If your job is stressful, the effects may be emotional, physical, and financial. If your finances are lagging, it may show as chaos in your physical environment and psycho-emotional stress. It's impossible to change one part of your life (wheel) without experiencing some sort of change rippling through the other parts.

Since the wheel is a metaphor for your life right now, take a good look at it again. Where are your thoughts going every day? Which areas of your life do you avoid dealing with and which areas hijack your energy in a negative direction? Which of those spokes do you know in your gut is draining or distracting you? Circle them. Even if they don't seem fitness related, these may be areas where your energy is being diverted, consciously or not, away from taking great care of yourself.

The way you think and feel, act and talk about these attention-sucking or energy-blocking areas are exactly the same way your body is experiencing them: as a drain. As science has demonstrated, everything is connected. And your thoughts and feelings are energy waves. So the way you think, feel, act, and even talk becomes the greater wave of you—a vibration—that precedes you and which you embody.

The life wheel exercise is merely a flashlight. It will help you to shine light on the areas of your consciousness, life, or habits that are covertly causing a disruption in your self-care. These are like covert circuit breakers, hidden energetic blocks that interfere with your self-care actions. If you have all the relevant information you need to make healthy choices and you're not making those choices, then there's something at work in your subconscious electrical panel that you need to shine the light on. If you want to change your actions, then you need to become aware of the thoughts or feelings that make you turn to food (or other avoidant behaviors) so you can effectively deal with them. Otherwise, you'll continue to fruitlessly fill your head with information and your tummy with potato chips. Becoming aware of your hidden energy blocks and dealing with them is the next step to rekindling your body relationship.

⌘ **Mental Fitness Exercise:** Segregate ten minutes a day to be dedicated solely toward your wellbeing. Put exercise, meditation, reading, a bubble bath—whatever is nurturing to you—into your daily schedule as of today.

⌘ **Mental Fitness Exercise:** Say "no!" to one thing in your schedule or life that impinges on your self-care time. Make a list of things you want to say no to but feel you can't. Then commit to saying no to one of those per week or month.

⌘ **Mental Fitness Exercise:** Do the Life Wheel exercise described in the body of this chapter.

Go to www.loveyourselffit.com/inspiration for a downloadable version of these exercises.

CHAPTER 7

The Home Wrecker: Fitness Ménage à Trois

"I love running. I'm not into marathons,
but I am into avoiding problems at an accelerated rate."

Jarod Kintz

I know, you probably read this chapter title and got really excited that a fitness philosophy was going to incorporate kinky sex! Sorry—it's not. Albeit there is a strong similarity in the subversive quality of a three-way affair on a relationship and what's subconsciously going on with your self-care, hence the name. But, this party isn't sexy! Bummer, I know. This is a deeper look at some barriers in your life that may be unknowingly sabotaging your self-care and ruining your relationship with your body and self-care. Getting past feminine philandering will allow you to take the time for this more personal round of clearing away blocks or viruses from your mindset.

In your fitness relationship you tend to unconsciously sabotage yourself with a three-way affair I call the fitness ménage à trois. Together tolerations, psycho-emotional needs, and coping mechanisms make up this adulterous triad. This three-way energy siphon is interwoven and feeds on itself to create a conspiracy that wreaks havoc on your self-care relationship every time.

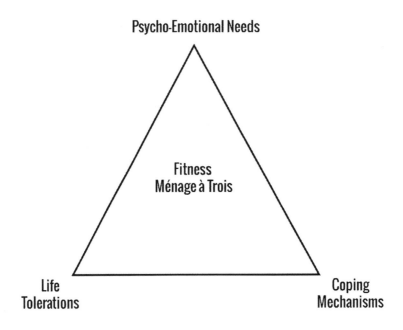

To best understand how the fitness ménage à trois functions to sabotage self-care, we'll use Samantha as an example. After completing the life wheel exercise, Samantha has determined her "body" spoke is frustrating her. She hates her body's appearance and struggles with keeping off excess weight (her toleration). She thinks she'll feel confident or loved (her psycho-emotional need) if she loses weight. Out of habit, frustration, and sometimes temptation, Samantha eats for reasons other than hunger or eats more than she's hungry for (her coping mechanism). Frustrated by her repeated attempts to lose weight, eat better, and start exercising, Samantha can't understand why she can't stick with a program.

Samantha is stuck in an unconscious, destructive battle with her needs, tolerations, and coping mechanisms, a.k.a. the fitness ménage à trois. These three elements are working together to ruin her relationship with her body and keep her in a vicious cycle of fitness failure. Samantha's weight is a toleration, because her thoughts about her body provoke negative feelings. She also has an unmet psycho-emotional need for love that's contributing to her displeasure with her body. Samantha believes her value, hence lovability, is based on being beautiful. Because of this she's trying to meet this need for love—to feel better about herself—by changing her body. She thinks she'll feel confident and valuable if she becomes more beautiful (in our culture: thin). The way she copes with these (her unmet psycho-emotional need and unresolved toleration) is with food. Eating is her coping mechanism. Her coping mechanism is exacerbating her weight toleration and delaying a healthful resolution of her needs. This intangible trio has made her feel unhealthy, disempowered, and frustrated. Fitness ménage à trois in full swing, Samantha is stuck in a vicious, relationship-ruining cycle which she won't break free of until she addresses this triad.

Can you sympathize with Samantha's struggles? If you're female, you can likely relate to her experience. Most women feel, or have felt, exactly the same way and run the same vicious gauntlet Sam has: tolerating your weight, wanting to change, and sabotaging yourself with food. Repeat.

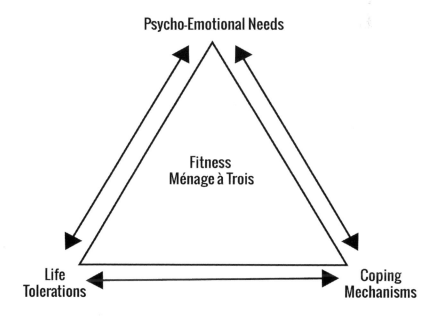

Psycho-emotional needs—or needy thinking—is often the source of tolerations and coping mechanisms. As is apparent in Samantha's story, each element in the fitness ménage à trois affects or aggravates the other two. But there's good news: you're not powerless over this party! They're each born of mind. They're a thought, a belief, and a feeling and therefore all fluid and changeable, just like your mind.

Be it the ill-fitting size six pants in your closet which you tolerate daily, a need-based, never ending battle to be thin, or the cookie dough ice cream that helps you cope, you likely have some circuits to rewire.

The following section describes each home wrecker and offers some solutions.

Tolerations

Tolerations are the easiest place to start when it comes to the fitness ménage à trois. They stand out the most, because they're the parts of you or your life that are most obvious, or irritate you most. If you look at your life wheel again, you'll notice that the low-rated spokes are the areas of your life with tolerations. These tolerations are exactly what they sound like: things in your life that you're putting up with. They're elements of your life that remind you of what's incomplete, damaged, or missing altogether. Some are large and some are small, but they all stimulate negative thoughts or feelings and usually drain your energy.

Most of us have tolerations in our physical environments: an ugly nick in the drawer of the nightstand, an overdue oil change on the car, or a closet filled with three different sizes of clothes. Less concrete and possibly more disruptive life tolerations can be found in areas other than one's environment. For example, a coworker who takes credit for your work, a marriage that's stressful, or the twenty pounds you've been trying to lose for five years. Life tolerations can be things you've been biting your tongue about or issues you try desperately to ignore. They can be feelings, a state of mind, a set of bad habits, lack of boundaries, or your own denial.

Each toleration drains your energy, because it sparks a line of thinking that's negative and draining. Tolerations allow you to "should" on yourself. That's right, you're shoulding on yourself. You believe you're stuck with this thing the way it is, because you lack the time, energy, or money to fix it. Simply put: tolerations reduce you to a limited, small, alone self or what's called the little-i. Your little-i is synonymous with the ego, or your most petty, needy self. You *should* fix the nightstand, but you don't have time. You s*hould* get the car tuned up, but you don't have the money. You *should* talk to your boss about your coworker, but you lack the confidence. You look at your closet stuffed with ill-fitting clothes of three sizes, and you feel guilty—you *should* lose weight. If you let them, tolerations hijack your thinking and whisper to you of not being, doing, or having enough. Tolerations drain your energy and derail the positive and creative thoughts, feelings, and energy you could be putting into your self-care.

What do we do about them? We clear them up! Most tolerations require a bi-fold solution: a shift in perception and a physical step, setting a boundary, or making a move toward resolution. Once you shift the way you perceive a situation, person, or event it often is no longer a toleration. Shifting your energy and thoughts can help you. Shifting your perspective means pulling your tolerations out of the limited little-i realm, and moving them to the opposite, unlimited, anything is possible Big-I zone (which will be covered in Chapter 10). How can it help? Let's see: do the taxes in a foul mood, or be in a decent or peaceful mind-state and do the taxes? Which will suck less? Which state is most helpful, efficient, and creative? (If you can't wait, Chapter 14 *Shifting Your Perceptions*, offers several tools to help change your perspective.)

New thoughts create different actions, so decide to change your mind.

Shift your thoughts and take back the siphoning of your energy. Wouldn't it be great if you could think and feel any way you choose to about every person, situation, and thing on this planet? Politics, the environment, your boss, your family, you name it, are all held in your conscious reality however you would like it to be. Oh wait, you can choose your thoughts. Reclaim your cognitive ground, girl! You're the only one who can redirect your thinking, feelings, and perceptions. And redirecting your thoughts about your body, food, and exercise is exactly the habit that will shift your self-care from difficult to easy. You don't have to have a huge, therapist-involved session. You simply decide to think differently. Whatever your crappy thought, decide it's bullshit and pick a different, true thought that is more aligned with the experience you desire. You free yourself from a toleration or negative thought not by obsessing on it, but by picking up something else with your mind—an alternate, equally true and better-feeling thought. Then ask for guidance, love, or help from your highest self, God, or spirit—whatever you choose to call it.

It might sound Pollyanna-ish or like a major endeavor, but it really is only a small series of conscious choices. You're always the one in charge of your thoughts. Take, for example, my bathroom breakdown. One Saturday afternoon I was digesting a bad medical report, PMS-ing, fighting with my spouse, and dealing with two moody, whiney four- and six-year old children. I was in emotional hell inside and remember feeling as if I were going to explode with rage or tears. I excused myself to the bathroom and shut the door. I sat on the toilet seat and started to cry. Then it suddenly hit me: I could change my thoughts! I mean, I had studied all this stuff for years, and this was one of those moments to use what I knew in my head but not in my heart (yet): it was within my power to steer my thoughts in the opposite direction.

By this time my four-year-old was at the door pounding on it and crying "Mommeee!" I closed my eyes and said, "I'm not sitting in this. I can shift and glide through this shit. I'm asking for Grace and Divine

Guidance. I'm going to allow the part of me that knows better to run this right now." I said a little prayer and it was as if someone poured a bucket of ice water on my head—I woke up. I felt refreshed and strangely non-attached to these events that a moment ago seemed to suck me into a vortex of crushing emotion. I immediately felt like: "I can do this."

My daughter had stopped crying and was in my husband's arms outside the bathroom door when I opened it. "Are you okay?" he asked, looking at me funny. "Yep! I'm okay," I said and thanked him. I took my daughter into my arms and told her it was okay too. My kids immediately calmed, and we all went about our day. I went from a puddle of goo to clear and slightly optimistic with one small choice and a dose of the divine.

It seems so massive when you are feeling overwhelmed, because you get sucked into the emotion. But in the midst of any emotion you always retain your power of choice. You can choose a different direction with your energy or actions, especially when you ask for help.

Changing the way you're thinking about your boss, or exercise, or your dinged fender starts with a teeny, tiny decision. Then another. And another. It's not always easy at first, but it will become so with practice. If your boss is an asshole, decide to find something redeeming about him (or the office, or your desk) and focus solely on that. Then when the thought "What an asshole!" comes back, go again to the redeeming thought. Do the same with exercise or your car. There's no room for a shift in consciousness until you decide you want one. There's no one who can shift you but you. The decision to shift isn't one giant leap; it's small, repetitive redirection choices you make all day about the hardest things and thoughts, like tolerations.

Byron Katie's "The Work" has worked in my life (and for many of my clients). She offers a four-question technique for resolving errant thinking. The Work seeks to instigate the disturbing thoughts that are inciting bad feelings and asks the user to question those thoughts and then find the truth in their opposite thoughts. Using her book or CD set *"Loving What Is"* (or visit www.thework.com) will allow you to experience, hear, or see, The Work in progress. The live recordings do it better justice than I can on paper. So I strongly encourage you to check out The Work for yourself.

The second part of clearing up tolerations is the physical element: boundary, baby step, or move in a different direction. This means coping with lower-rated spokes using creative solutions and clear boundaries.

Let's pretend you have children, a full-time career, stress is your copilot, and "I don't have time!" is your mantra. Both your body and relationship spokes are rated low. You want to lose fifteen pounds and spend more time with your kids.

How can these spokes be dealt with effectively and creatively using baby steps? Let your mind wander. Meditate. Pray. Ask friends, family, or coworkers for ideas. Can you take your kids for a walk every night after dinner? Could your family go to the park on the weekends and play a game or group sport? How about getting your children involved in a new family project? For example, "Project HY: Healthy & Yummy" is one that focuses on shopping and preparing healthy, yummy snacks and meals. Put the kids online to do research, get them to pick recipes out of cookbooks and magazines, or take them shopping and have a contest to see who can pick or help cook the best tasting, healthiest item based on food labels. By taking on Project HY, you and your kids would be learning more about foods, eating healthier, and spending additional time interacting with each other. Two spokes, one stone.

Strengthening a spoke of your life can also be a commitment to yourself. You might sign up for a new gym membership or order fish and veggies instead of a meatball sub. A messy garage might beg a weekend to clean and organize. The areas of your life that are thanklessly draining your energy and sidetracking your thinking are the ones that most need clearing up.

Occasionally, clearing up a toleration is more involved, leading to permanent changes in your life. Contacting a financial planner for your lagging finances, sitting down with a child to have the discussion you've been dreading, or choosing to spend less time with a negative person are examples of physical actions to clean up your life wheel and resolve your tolerations.

You've probably resolved many tolerations throughout your lifetime by creating environments that supported you or eliminated a toleration. For example, in college your goal was better grades, so you joined a study group, sought tutoring, and limited your partying to weekends. If you think about it, there's probably some way in which you've shifted yourself or your life by making tiny steps to change your mind, environment, or actions. You redirected your thoughts and energy, and you took action to create a different reality.

Tolerations are easy to handle when your psycho-emotional needs aren't fueling them.

Psycho-emotional Needs

The psycho-emotional wellbeing spoke may be the most crucial and powerful spoke in your life wheel when it comes to your behaviors. Your perceptions, thoughts, and feelings about the world color how you interpret the rest of your spokes and your life as a whole.

I view psycho-emotional needs as part your personality or wiring, and part conditioning or elements that have been developed within you as you've moved through life. When met in healthy ways, psycho-emotional needs are sedate and passive gifts that contribute to your life. The need to be creative is undeniably an asset to a marketing executive or a driving force for an interior designer. However, if a need is unmet and unquestioned, it can be disruptive, wreaking havoc upon relationships, careers, or physical wellbeing.

For instance, the need to be creative could be problematic in a person's life if she had no outlet for her ingenuity. She might amuse herself by inventing negative stories about neighbors, or boredom could entice her to devise a way to steal from her employer. It's best to identify and meet psycho-emotional needs in healthy ways.

I'm sure you're doing your best to meet your needs right now, healthfully or un-healthfully, consciously or unconsciously. Because of this subconscious element, your internal needs may motivate you to behave in ways you're not aware of or have a hard time controlling. Like Samantha, if your need to be nurtured is not being met, you could be undermining your health by overeating. Seeking pleasure when really you want nurturing is commonplace. With a little insight, you can look at your coping mechanisms (like eating) for a clue as to what you need psycho-emotionally and aren't getting.

Any coping mechanism you use regularly can help identify your needs. If you had to guess, what would you say is your internal catalyst for turning to food? Think about your normal overeating routine. What are you wanting when you turn to food? Nurturing? Reward? Revenge? Pleasure? Fulfillment? Human touch? Write down what you know or believe could be motivating your behavior. Finding the internal catalyst for turning to food, or any detrimental behavior, is the first step to freeing yourself from it.

Tolerations are drivers for psycho-emotional needs as well. For myself, unfinished house projects irritate me (tolerations). So I feel burdened by the feeling of incompletion. My stressful thought of "I need to finish all my projects in order to relax and enjoy my house" is nutty and not conducive to a happy life at home. These thoughts and feelings point to my psycho-emotional needs for completion and freedom. I believe I must complete all tasks or responsibilities before I allow myself to relax (freedom). My need for completion or freedom will drive me to stay up late, or overschedule myself to weed the planter, or touch up paint in the hallway. Is it true that my house is not enjoyable until it's "finished"? Of course not! It's fine, and moreover, that belief system will stress me out and not allow me to relax in my own home. Houses are never "finished". But let's stay focused on your insanity right now, not mine!

Use your top three tolerations to identify your needs. Once you've identified them, you'll want to address them. There are lots of ways to go about doing this. You can find a skilled coach or a trained therapist, or try a book on a quick therapy, like EFT. These needs don't in and of themselves demand therapy as they are generally not life-wreckers. However, they are disruptive and can lead to destructive behaviors (like overeating), therefore beg your attention.

I've found that the influence of psycho-emotional needs lessened as I've cleaned up my unresolved issues. (I know I said we needed to focus on your insanity, but let's go back to mine for a moment.) My need for "completed house projects" has become smaller and smaller as I've used the CORE technique (I'll explain this in a moment) to process my unresolved feelings about my insecurities, judgments, and perfectionism. Now I sit typing—six days before Thanksgiving Day—with my Halloween décor in a pile in my garage. Silly to you perhaps, but a monumental shift for me! Addressing my need to have my house projects "complete" I can now prioritize my energy and attention so I can choose to let the plastic pumpkins and ghoul napkins sit for three more days. Five years ago I would have been compelled to organize and store the décor before I sat to write. Now I have the choice, because my need is not driving my behavior.

Like an old crack in your windshield, unresolved psycho-emotional stuff—needs—make it hard to see the road you're currently driving upon clearly. If we were girlfriends chatting over a cup of tea, I would suggest you use the CORE technique. If I were coaching you, I'd take you through it. You can use the CORE for any number of things: relationship issues, insecurities, judgments, and even childhood hurts. It's simple, fast, and like its acronym, cuts to the core of the issues energy-wise. Tom Stone of Great Life Technologies has created multiple ways, he calls them the Pure Awareness Techniques, to deal with emotions. Some techniques ask you to become conscious of the feeling in your body. Stone, like Byron Katie, has written several books, but my favorite is *The Power of How*. One method, which he calls the "CORE technique", requires you to be mentally aware of an emotion as a physical presence in your body. You can try it right now.

Sit alone quietly and recall a situation that was really emotionally upsetting to you. Were you jealous, angry, or sad? Once you have a grasp of the situation, close your eyes. Ask yourself if you feel this emotion anywhere in your body. Await a noticeable sensation in your body. This sensation can manifest anywhere, such as energy that feels like a tightness in your stomach or an ache in your chest. Once located, focus all your attention there. Imagine you have to describe the sensation to a doctor. Feel it, visualize it, put your attention into the center of it; focus on it totally. If your mind wanders, bring it back to the sensation in your body.

Find the nucleus, the core, the very center where the sensation seems most concentrated. It helps to imagine this core looking like a satellite view of a hurricane. Keep bringing your attention to the center or pinpoint of the sensation. Sometimes I have my clients or even my kids imagine they're sliding, roller skating, or surfing down that hurricane core or eye. Keep moving down the center of this hurricane until the feeling disappears. If it moves to a different part of your body, just follow it. Keep focusing on the eye until there's no sensation left. You may need to repeat the technique if you still feel a physical sensation. When the process is complete, you will feel a relief of the original physical sensation and an emotional sense of "ah" or relief.

In the end, you should be able to recall the situation that originally upset you without feeling overwhelmed. You will feel neutral. The CORE technique helps dissolve the angst around feeling an emotion or the childlike fear built up about experiencing emotion. I find it often relieves the negative emotion altogether. You, as the emotionally mature adult you are, will become able to feel the emotion without being overwhelmed or sucked into it.

The CORE technique can be challenging at first, particularly if you're unaccustomed to working on your mindset. But it's an effective and quick remedy *you can do on your own.* As with anything, it gets easier with practice and takes less time to resolve your feelings. Again, I highly recommend you hear a sample of Tom's techniques live. (Visit http://thepowerofhow. com/CORE.html for audio samples.)

This is a tool to remove the sabotaging programming running in the background of your mind. And it won't do anything for you unless you use it! Your programming is nothing to be afraid of or worthy of self-condemnation. Be open to looking at it and determining what's derailing you. Upgrade your MBSL software for free!

Coping Mechanisms

From the time you were a child, you've probably had negative feelings arise that were sometimes overpowering. For a child, overwhelming feelings can be terrifying. When you started having negative feelings, you weren't aware of what they were or what was happening inside of you. All you knew was that the experience was traumatic and you were too small to throw darts at people's heads. Even for an adult, feelings can be overinflated, uncomfortable, or painful. It was probably quite scary from a child's perspective to think that the way you felt in a given moment was out of your control or might not go away. So you adapted to negative feelings by teaching yourself how to *not* feel them. You developed coping mechanisms to help yourself survive psychologically.

Few individuals learn how to feel a feeling, honor it, and then let it pass in a healthy way. The way you learned to feel or avoid emotions as a child is often the same way you're handling your feelings today. If you learned that a tantrum relieved your feelings because it changed the behavior of your caregivers, then you probably still practice tantrum-like behavior when you start to feel a negative emotion. You might break down crying when a conversation leads to a sensitive area, or you may fly into a rage when you feel a boundary crossed. As an adult you have the mental and emotional capacity to feel your feelings fully, though you may still be operating as if you were a child emotionally.

Coping mechanisms are the methods you use to avoid your feelings or to attempt to meet your psycho-emotional needs. They're an empty shell of temporary relief found in a substance or behavior. Because coping mechanisms are things you do to avoid or distract yourself, they sabotage your goals and often create more tolerations.

You use a coping mechanism in an attempt to change your thoughts and feelings superficially. It can be a physical addiction to painkillers or a thought pattern of being worried. They can also be lifestyle habits like always having too much on your plate. They help you avoid a situation in your life that seems challenging to resolve or you fear you can't deal with.

Be they small or large, life altering or merely inconvenient, coping mechanisms are often addictions. If you have a couple martinis, perhaps you can avoid feeling stressed about your mortgage. If you binge on chocolate chip cookies, maybe you can distract yourself from the loneliness you're feeling. The excitement you'll get rolling dice all night in Las Vegas might numb your anger towards your husband. Martinis, cookies, and craps are not inherently evil, but they become destructive when your mindset is motivated by a need-based, insatiable state that runs deeper than modest enjoyment or periodic entertainment.

Whether it's the bad habit you just can't seem to kick, or the New Year's resolution you can never keep, you often strive to stop using a coping mechanism without addressing the mindset (thoughts, beliefs, or feelings) that's driving it. As you've done with fitness pursuits in the past, you try to mimic a behavior without shifting the mind to match. This is like undertaking a mathematical equation on your computer without loading the appropriate math program into the hard drive. You can do the equation, but it will be "by hand"—the same way you can force yourself into mimicking a fitness routine or temporarily avoiding the Oreos.

Gary Zukav in his book *The Seat of the Soul* talks about the spiritual gains you make when you resist an addiction. He says you get closer to your own spirit, your authentic power, when you resist an addiction. Conversely, indulgence pulls you away from your highest self. Zukav claims that each time you resist, you take a step closer to spirit and grow a bit stronger in the skill of resisting temptations the next time you're faced with them.

If your coping mechanisms are mind-altering habits like alcohol or pills, then obviously you have to abstain and/or seek professional help to resolve them. Serious physical and chemical addictions will most likely require professional help. Otherwise, you can start reining in your coping mechanisms immediately. (By the way, cookie addiction is not as serious.)

I'm not suggesting you have to go through your entire closet of issues from childhood to present day to find peace with food and show up for exercise. But I am saying you have to address the feelings and thoughts that are interfering with your know-do equation or pulling you off-center. It doesn't matter what the "virus" running in your mental background is made up of—tolerations, needs, coping mechanisms, or a lack of boundaries. If they have a virus-like way of interfering with your desired programming (goals), or you can't figure out why you always sabotage yourself, it's worth running a mental virus scan. Without addressing the emotions involved in your avoidance, you'll stay stuck or you'll simply find another addiction, transferring from alcohol to cigarettes, food to work, or sex to gambling. Coping mechanisms are interchangeable when the source is unresolved.

Get professional help if you're dealing with something beyond the scope of this book.

⌘ **Mental Fitness Exercise:** Use your life wheel to make a list of your tolerations, five-ten max. Start with your most annoying two. Decide how you would like to think, feel, and act toward each toleration. What's the energy you'd like to have on the topic? Ask yourself if there's a mind shift, boundary to set, or decision to be made. Take baby steps in actions or thought redirection; one at a time to deal with them.

⌘ **Mental Fitness Exercise:** What are you using as coping mechanisms? When do you think you need them? Use Stone's or Katie's techniques to investigate or resolve them. Is there a connection between your tolerations, needs, and coping mechanisms?

🖱 Go to www.loveyourselffit.com/inspiration for a downloadable version of these exercises.

CHAPTER 8

Communication Skills 101: Listening

"No one is as deaf as the man who will not listen."
Jewish Proverb

I
n the last chapter we talked about the aspects of your life that influence your choices. The next part of connecting with your body is developing good communication skills, including discerning between physical and psycho-emotional cues.

Have you ever felt unheard by a sibling or child? Has your partner ever disregarded your feelings? Has a coworker completely ignored your request? Not being heard can be frustrating and hurtful, and with consistency it can be a deal breaker for a LTR. If you imagine building your self-care relationship with your body on the same principles you would a marriage, then good communication skills—listening and responding genuinely and appropriately—enhance and build the relationship. Naturally, poor communication skills, such as not listening and inflated reactions undermine and tear down a relationship. Reconnecting with your body means learning the essentials of conscious body-mind communication; this is the start of being nice to yourself!

Food, Eating, and Emotions

Food is a loaded subject! It's a topic that carries a ton of shoulds, emotions, and confusion for many people. Not surprisingly we use food for a multitude of reasons other than physical sustenance. "What's physical sustenance?" you ask. I know it's a foreign concept for many Americans, but originally food was invented for physical nourishment and growth, not as a taste bud vibrator.

Women think about food, weight, bodies, and all related topics every day—sometimes throughout the entire day—but we pretend it's not an issue. We don't *talk* about it nearly as much as we *think* about it. Sometimes we may make passive comments or jokes about ourselves without really surfacing the pungency of the thoughts and feelings we're having. It's mildly reminiscent of the way women used to avoid the subject of sex or being sexually harassed: body, shame, and insecurity tied together beget immobility and secrecy.

Many people believe that certain foods are addictive, our serving sizes are too big, or our food is over processed, and that one or more of these are the cause of our societal obesity and overindulgence. Though these are contributive, I don't believe they're fully responsible for our standard of overeating. When it comes to eating too much, I believe it's a person's mental-emotional state and lack of body awareness that are the primary culprits. Therefore, I'm not going to address what we eat with a list of good or bad foods, or even offer recipes in the back of the book. I am going to address why we eat and how to alter our internal environment with food.

In American culture, many of us eat for reasons other than physical hunger. Often undiagnosed, low-level eating disorders are commonplace and even socially acceptable. We're so immersed in our off-balanced eating habits that many of us don't realize how askew our "normal" eating is.

There are numerous reasons why so many of us overeat. Food is plentiful in countries like ours, and eating has become more entertainment than survival mechanism. We eat for just about every social and business occasion; whenever we gather, we eat. Cooking is regarded as an art form, with entire networks and social clubs dedicated to the culinary arts. We're surrounded and bombarded by food smells, sights, and sounds on a daily basis. We're enticed by giant billboards, TV ads, magazines, radio ads, samples, and larger-than-ever portions.

Many circumstances stimulate you to eat. From childhood you likely followed a feeding schedule set by your parents or school, and later your workplace. You were *not taught how to listen to your body* or how to figure out what to eat and when. Proper eating was dictated to you. Certain foods were "good", others were "bad", and most foods had their right time of day to be served. Some of us grew up with less food, food manipulation or games, or perhaps parents with eating or body issues, all of which made eating and food more emotionally charged. It's no wonder that most people are unable or don't bother to differentiate between physiological hunger, emotional hunger, and conditioned responses.

Though conditioning is part of our overeating problem, the biggest factor is our inability to distinguish between physical and emotional hunger. We often eat for psychological or emotional reasons. Food cravings, compulsive overeating, and clinical eating disorders like bulimia are addictions to unbalanced eating or bingeing on food, usually with some sort of compensatory behavior. Some are deadly, others just misery makers, but none of these disorders are really about food. They're attempts to avoid or control a feeling, distract from a perceived reality, or fill an empty emotional place—all coping mechanisms to deal with uncomfortable emotions.

Food is used in all kinds of ways. Sometimes you experience some sort of discomfort, restlessness, or perhaps boredom and you try to distract or reward yourself by eating. Other times you try to cope with anger, pain, or depression by eating. You also eat as a reward or to celebrate. For some the act of eating is like sex: it's the only physical pleasure that's safe and enjoyable. Eating may be the only way an individual will allow herself to receive, indulge, or be nurtured. It is said that food is medicine, but that doesn't mean it's an OTC drug for heartbreak or warped thinking.

You know this: emotional hunger will never be satisfied with food. "If eating hasn't worked for you yet, it never will!" Food will never fulfill you; it will only fill your stomach. Because overeating is not a sustenance issue, it must be treated on the psychological, emotional, and spiritual level. Emotional overeating is hunger from a deep part of the self, so that's where you look for a solution: the deepest part of yourself. Don't get scared; you won't bite you.

Differentiating between emotional, conditioned, and physical hunger begins with recognizing your personal patterns, habits, and triggers. Start by keeping notes via your cell phone or paper to observe when, where, and why you're overeating or eating for reasons other than physical hunger. Record your trigger points, be they a time of day, an activity (or the cessation thereof), or even a place. Notice if when you come home from work, finish your work, or walk into your office you may be triggered to eat. Recognizing when you're triggered will help you become aware of what you were experiencing (internally or externally) before you chose food, instead of dealing with your feelings or listening to your body.

In your note taking, investigate which circumstances are triggering you. Which feelings or thoughts are you experiencing when you want to eat? Is there a recurring theme of situations or emotions when you turn to food? It's not atypical for a person to eat in a healthy way (or not eat) all day and return home at night to binge. If the coping mechanism section didn't help you fully clarify the roots of your overeating, then investigation will help you uncover what's behind the food-mood connection for you.

Once you identify the triggers or situations that provoke overeating, you can attend to the thoughts and feelings that inspire your behavior. If you find you have one or more environmental provocateurs, change your experience in that environment with a break in your habitual behavior. Plot and execute a different physical or environmental response than usual, such as skip in your front door instead of walking, have tea instead of ice cream after dinner, or bring trail mix instead of cookies to the office.

Internal shifters will be the most powerful to change your behavior and energy with food. You can use the techniques you learned in the last chapter (CORE or The Work) to resolve your remaining psycho-emotional drivers. Additionally, the next two sections of this chapter deal with understanding emotions and enhancing your perspective of feelings, both physically and psychologically. In other words, learn to deal with your feelings before you wash them down with a giant batch of chocolate chip cookies. Read on, milady, read on.

Emotions—How do I not swallow them?

Dealing with feelings (a.k.a. emotions) means you stop seeing them as that crazy, drunk uncle you just want to avoid at Thanksgiving and instead start to view them as gifts. "How the hell can I think of that crazy drunk as a gift?" you ask. I know it's a leap, but if you think about it, your emotions have been a best friend to you—unafraid to be honest with you about the state of your life or relationships. Because emotions are deeply interwoven with your thoughts and physiology, they can teach you about yourself, your boundaries, and your relationships with others. Your feelings can be intuitive and offer guidance. I like to think of emotions as an alarm system. Feelings let you know when something is awry in your inner or outer world. They'll be honest with you when something isn't right, a boundary has been crossed, or the current situation is out of alignment with who you are. They'll tell you directly that your thoughts are out of alignment with your highest self. In this light, they're a gift.

Dealing with emotions can be uncomfortable. Often times your fear and aversion to small amounts of discomfort are the cause of your inability to cope with feelings. You may have conditioned yourself to be so intolerant of discomfort that you confuse it with pain. Discomfort is not pain, and it won't hurt you or me. Discomfort is merely uncomfortable. It's only an unpleasant experience and one you and anyone can handle.

Though we often avoid it, the ability to experience discomfort often brings success, reward, or gratification. Enduring graduate school, working overtime on a project, and sticking to a course of therapy are all examples of uncomfortable situations that, when tolerated, will reap rewards. Sometimes growth means making uncomfortable decisions: like signing up for a mortgage payment, putting your child into drug rehab, or for some of us eating our veggies. When it comes to growing up and shifting your mindset, get comfortable with being uncomfortable so you can learn to experience, resolve, and release stale ways of being.

Consciously choosing to be temporarily uncomfortable to resolve an issue or grow stronger is very different than living in denial in Toleration City. Tolerations are a form of not dealing with the reality of your thoughts, story, or a situation. Discomfort during reality shifts is like teething or growing pains: optimal and necessary.

Cognitive behavioral therapy (CBT) is the best-known method of dealing with difficult emotions. CBT can be extremely valuable with the right therapist, but I've experienced amazing results with other techniques and modalities like the CORE, The Work, and brief therapies.

As PNI and like research have revealed, your feelings live in your body as well as your heart and mind. Present feelings and past stored emotions are burned into your psyche and body via a complex network of nervous and chemical connections. Extreme emotional traumas are seared even deeper.

Some practitioners of psychology believe that if feelings are to be fully resolved, one must pursue a therapy that's inclusive of physiology. The idea being that our bodies store feelings physically, and therefore the most effective way to process them is through the body. EMDR (Eye Movement Desensitization and Reprocessing) and EFT (Emotional Freedom Technique) are several newer therapy models that include your body in the therapy process. These psycho-physiological therapies are referred to as quick or brief therapies since they work quicker than conventional therapies (in less than 15 sessions). Though the science on the later (EFT) is less abundant, it's picking up steam in the arena of appetitive disorders. Moreover, you can do it yourself, it's practically free, and it would certainly do you no harm. In contrast, EMDR is highly researched and positively regarded for trauma and post-traumatic stress disorder. On that note, I do recommend them, but their instruction is above my pay grade at present. I recommend instruction from a professional trained or licensed in the modality.

Because emotion is part physiological, breath work is another method to help you deal with negative emotions. Deep controlled breathing is a staple of many relaxation techniques, yoga, and meditation, all of which help calm emotions. Specific types of breathing stimulate the Vagus Nerve which is the part of your nervous system that calms you post fight-or-flight response. More data is revealing the drug-like effects of deep breathing and chanting (rhythmic sounds) on the part of the brain that controls emotion and elevates mood.[6]

Be patient with yourself. Remember Rome wasn't built in a day—few things of quality are—and neither will be your new LTR with your body. This LTR is a process made up of small steps. As in the dating world, you may "fall" for someone on the first date but that does not a relationship make! It will take time to learn how to honor your emotions and deal with them without fear or dismissal instead of eating. There are many other resources available to help you learn more about emotions and managing them healthfully. If you need to, please seek resources beyond this book for the how-to's of emotional management.

⌘ **Mental Fitness Exercise:** Start taking notes on your eating. Notice when, where, and why you're triggered to want to overeat—your internal and external triggers. Hone your differentiating skills. Clarify your internal and external shifters and be creative about solutions (shifters).

⌘ **Mental Fitness Exercise:** Try some new quick therapy techniques with a licensed practitioner: EFT, EMDR, breath work, or traditional CBT.

Go to www.loveyourselffit.com/inspiration for a downloadable version of these exercises.

Developing Listening Skills

If you've ever been to therapy you know one of the first issues you start working on is listening. "Lisa, did you hear what Doug said?" And the therapist starts to teach you how to actively listen. Learning how to listen to your body is an active process as well, and absolutely crucial to learning to be at peace with food, your body, and weight.

Once you understand the internal or environmental triggers of over-eating, you can focus on developing better physical listening skills. Be it eating, sleeping, or movement there are two common ways people are deaf and disregard the messages they get from their bodies: conscious and unconscious.

Shelby is unconscious. She eats without awareness. Usually in a hurry, you'll find her eating on the run, in the car, or in front of the television.

She might talk throughout entire meals, nibbling away until everything on her plate has disappeared. Shelby is the type of eater who won't remember what her food tastes like after the first bite and may be alarmed at how much she's actually consumed. She's a professional at tuning out and a bit of a feminine philanderer.

Rebecca, on the other hand, is conscious. She's aware of what and how she's eating, even though she's not really present while eating either. She's the type of eater who deliberately eats when she's not hungry and often binges. Unlike the unconscious eater, she spends time on food. Rebecca may proclaim her love for food or cooking. In fact, to her food is like a lover. Though passionate, she's often ashamed of her food-related behaviors and will hide the amount she eats. Rebecca is aware she has a problem with overeating but doesn't want to admit the depth to which she's using food.

Both Shelby and Rebecca are deaf; neither is listening or responding appropriately to her body. Can you relate to either?

If either is to learn to listen, she must acknowledge her behavior. For the unconscious eater, Shelby, this means becoming aware of the way she's eating; she must slow down enough to be conscious and listen. While the conscious eater, Rebecca, may be aware of her eating, she must become willing to connect with and feel her body in order to address her reasons for overeating.

Listening to your body is challenging at first. There are many reasons why people don't listen to their bodies: distraction, feminine philandering, errant thinking, or ignorance. Whatever the cause, the solution requires you to pay attention to your physical self. Like Shelby and Rebecca, this means becoming conscious and willing to be in your body. Being present *in* your body is simply being aware of and attentive to your physical messages.

Hearing your body's cues at first might seem somewhat foreign. But understand that your body has never stopped talking to you. It has been telling you what it wants and needs your entire life. Communication between your conscious mind and your physical body is innate—you have only to clear away the cobwebs and distractions, and listen.

The toughest part of listening physically is filtering out the distractions—not letting your thoughts, emotions, or environment interfere with your communication and choices. Once you've handled the internal distractions (some of which you learned about in the previous section), listening to your body is much easier. Think of listening to your body as if you are modeling listening behavior for your spouse—the actual person. You want him to listen, don't you? Would you want him to listen to you only when it comes to mowing the lawn? Or would you like him to hear and respond to your requests about the garbage, putting the seat down, and picking up his socks too? Start listening to all of your body's signals. Listen to it the way you want others to listen to you. Being tired or sore, having a headache, or being thirsty are all strong signals your body will send you. Truly hearing your body's signals means first acknowledging the message (okay, I hear you), then honoring your body's request (okay, I'll take care of that). When you are tired you sleep, nap, or rest. Sore? Get a massage or take a hot bath. And so forth. Follow through on your body's requests, because your physical state of being greatly affects your mental state of being and your ability to listen to satiation cues.

Listening is also more difficult when you're preoccupied with environmental distractions. People, phone, radio, computer, TV, driving, working, or anything else that begs your attention will take it from your body if you allow it. At first, tuning in to your body's voice may require you to minimize or eliminate the distractions in your environment, especially before or during eating. Support yourself with distraction-free zones initially. If you were starting a discussion with your spouse or boss, you would turn off the TV or take your ear buds out to listen, particularly if the topic was feelings or dinner plans! Do the same for your body. It takes less than a minute to get tuned in, and once you master listening without external distractions, you'll eventually be able to listen to your body's messages anywhere—even at a three-ring circus.

Start a dialogue with your body. Get in the habit of asking your body if it's physically hungry for food or wanting something else. Does it want touch? Massage? Sex? Relaxation? Sleep? Movement? A drink (of water, you lush)? When you're really listening, you'll get clear physical cues of what your body wants—either a physical sensation in your body or an intuition. Other times it will seem like a fleeting thought. The more you practice listening to your body, knowing it's always talking to you, the better you'll get at interpreting its requests.

If you know anyone who's good at listening to her body, interview that person. Ask her what she does or says to herself when she knows she's full. How does she handle situations in which she's not physically hungry but there's a large spread of enticing and decadent food? Don't let her answer, "I just don't eat it." Ask her about her self-talk. "Spill it bitch!" has worked for me in the past. What does she say to herself when she feels tempted? How does she know her body has had enough, and how does she listen to it when she's deep in conversation or busy? Use your resources to help you find solutions and listen more attentively.

Try this exercise when you're starting the listening process. Get yourself alone and in a quiet environment. Make sure you're not ravenous, but just slightly hungry, and ask your body what it really wants to eat: sweet, salty, savory, sour, crunchy, creamy, soft, cold, hot, or any other adjectives you enjoy. Don't restrict yourself based on "good" or "bad" foods. Notice the first food that comes to mind. Be as specific as possible about what your body wants. Once you two decide, put the food on your tongue for a minute or so, and just let it sit there. Savor the flavor in your mouth. Take your time eating the food as slowly as possible without distraction.

Let yourself chew, swallow, and pause before taking another bite. The more focused on the food and eating process you are, the better you'll hear your body's signals. Some call this "conscious eating" or "mindful eating". Conscious eating is the only way to fly when you're learning to listen to your body.

By the way, bingeing isn't loving food. Where's the love in a quickie-orgy? Or did I miss that in the Kamasutra and the Cooking Channel?

There are more resources to help you listen to your body. Conscious eating proponents offer plenty of suggestions and support to help you better tune in and experience eating. Some people numerically rate their hunger on a zero-to-ten scale and only eat past a certain number like five or six. Others have found success in external support. Joining a twelve-step program or support group, or seeing a therapist can be great catalysts. For many, asking for guidance from an inner or higher power, or relying on meditation and/or prayer helps immensely.

As I learned to listen, I found that the more consciously I moved my body, the more of a connection I made. Yoga improved my hearing. It became easier for me to listen and hear my body's messages. The more aware of your body you become through movement, the more likely you are to recognize signals from it. Ask your body to help you. Activities that encourage listening like yoga, the Feldenkrais Method, Tai Chi, Qi Gong, or the Alexander Technique can be quite helpful. Connection and listening can start anywhere!

Heeding the wisdom of your body is a learning process you'll master with time. And once you begin the practice of listening and respecting your body signals, you'll feel an upward lift in your emotional and energy levels. You'll feel good and think well of your choices, because you'll know in your gut you're in sync, listening to, and respecting your body. Physically your energy will increase, because your body will immediately respond to improved care and feeding, and will probably get more rest. It gets easier to listen the longer you practice.

⌘ **Mental Fitness Exercise:** Start a dialogue with your body about what it's hungry for and begin the practice of conscious eating.

⌘ **Mental Fitness Exercise:** Compile a personal 4-Way Temptation Manager using the chart below. The 4-Way Temptation Manager attends to the multi-causal layers of eating: emotions, thoughts, environment, and physical cravings. The Treat(ment) takes into consideration all the parts of you that might be hungry—body, mind, heart, and spirit—and helps you design a Treat(ment) for each trigger as well as a plan to nurture your body. You create a design to satisfy whichever part of you might be hungry or your whole self simultaneously. This is a tool to help you develop a way to deal with your emotions and to learn to listen to your body.

The 4-Way Temptation Manager consists of the following:

1. Identify each reason, trigger, or situation that compels you to eat (for nonphysical reasons). When, what, and where?

2. Clarify what you're really wanting or needing from food, or the experience of eating in each situation. What are you feeling or really wanting?

3. Develop Treat(ment)... physical, mental, emotional, and spiritual to target the need or want and fulfill you instead of your tummy. What can you do for your spirit or heart instead of eat? How could you redirect your mind or energize your body?

Trigger Situation	True Want or Need	Treatment	
At home, at night, after dinner	Feel needy / want treat	Emotional	Vent / Friend / Paint?
		Mental	Journal / Call coach
		Spiritual	Pray / Meditate / Read
		Physical	Hot Bath / Tea / Breathe

Post or keep open access to your 4-Way Manager. Put a version in your purse or on your phone.

Go to www.loveyourselffit.com/inspiration for a downloadable version of these exercises.

SECTION III

Redirecting to Center:
Being True to You

CHAPTER 9

Alignment: Partnering with Wholeness

"Physical strength can never permanently withstand the impact of spiritual force."

Franklin D. Roosevelt

Thus far we've discussed how all the seemingly different parts of your life influence your self-care and fitness choices. The focus has been on understanding and identifying what's interfering with your body-mind connection or driving a wedge between you and good self-care.

This and the next two chapters move you toward divine inspiration or what I call Aligned fitness. Aligned fitness is self-care motivated from a place beyond the physical. It's exercise and eating innately inspired! Aligned fitness stems from your connection with your most powerful form of inspiration and most resonant type of guidance: your Authentic Self.

RV for the Soul

As a byproduct of the human condition and our busy lifestyles, we often forget that there's so much more thriving beneath our epidermis than the accountant, the dancer, the tycoon, the friend, the mom, or the sister. There is spirit, a higher being, a soul, a universal intelligence dwelling in these bodies.

Our body is the means by which we relate to the world and to part of who we are. Without it, we can't express our thoughts and emotions, our creativity, or our spirits. We can't learn, build, love, or give. We need a body; and our bodies become lifeless vessels without an alert mind and an infused spirit (soul). In this sense, the body is the carriage of the soul.

In a state of alignment, you allow your soul to sit in the driver's seat of the vehicle called "you". When soul is allowed to express through one's personality and body, this is the authentic self. Let your spirit drive and your body becomes the vessel in which the real you actualizes its destiny: your body is your spirit's RV.

The Power of Wholeness

If you pay attention you'll notice that all struggle occurs when one part of the whole is out of alignment with the other parts. It's true in politics, families, sports teams, and within you. Alignment is the integration of all the elements of your self and a truce in your self-care relationship. It's the declaration of peace with your body.

The times in my life when I really struggled with eating or exercise were when my actions and intentions were incongruent. My thoughts and feelings, or body and spirit, were each pulling in different directions. There were periods when I really wanted to lose weight, but part of me still had a need to use food as an emotional crutch or weight as protection. Yet I would feel my body's response was unjustified: "How could these backstabbing thighs of mine topographically shape themselves into lumpy mashed potatoes with the donuts and chips they're getting? Donuts are smooth damn it! Traitors." In reality, the entire "me" wasn't united behind the goal of weight loss; therefore, exercising or eating healthfully became a hopeless endeavor, because I would end up unconsciously sabotaging myself.

All of you, your whole being, must be in alignment with your intentions or you'll find yourself running in circles around your goals. Scattered and misaligned energy produces the same in its physical wake. Thus, the next step in your self-care relationship building is the integration or alignment of your whole self.

Ending your toils with eating, exercise, or any other area of your life will resolve once you're internally aligned. Being internally aligned means you're aware of and acting from the values of your authentic self. Often intangible, but highly meaningful, authentic values hold a powerful place in your internal makeup. Freedom, love, health, connection, discipline, and levity are all examples of values. When you become aware of and act on the values that originate from your authentic self, you'll emerge a force to be reckoned with. You become internally aligned which is super-powered-power. (You know the power you feel when you find the most dynamite outfit and adorable shoes? Well, more powerful than that!)

Some alignment has been hardwired for us by biology. Some is created through clarifying values. An example of hardwired and clear values is the rescue scenarios you'll occasionally see on the news: the man pulling a child out of a burning car or the little girl saving a woman from drowning. The hard wiring of adrenalin, and the authentic wiring of love, or the value of human life kicks in, and a 67-year-old man springs into action, or the child produces a feat of strength beyond her normal abilities. The outcome is the same with either: action. Be it conscious choice or involuntary reaction, when you're clear and aligned, you'll act without question or internal struggle. In alignment, you'll find the power to consistently act. You'll find the power of wholeness.

You may know someone like Andrea, who failed to maintain weight loss, because of the unresolved psycho-emotional issue of sexual abuse. This is not an uncommon occurrence. Andrea regains the hundred pounds she lost, because part of her is not in alignment with being thin. (To a sexual abuse victim, male sexual attraction can be perceived as predatory.) She feels threatened when men are sexually attracted to her. She may have busted her butt to get the weight off, only to find herself feeling more vulnerable or uncomfortable than ever. Consciously or not, the misaligned part within her begins to dismantle her achievement and sabotage her weight maintenance by overeating or making excuses not to exercise. She regains the weight she lost and starts beating herself up mentally. Guilt and frustration soon follow. "Hello darkness, my old friend…"

Andrea doesn't understand why she failed to maintain her regimen. Not recognizing what went wrong, she ends up feeling frustrated, incapable, and guilty. Not only has she physically "failed" at keeping the weight off, but her emotional fallout further drains her of resolve to find a healthy, fit lifestyle.

The part of Andrea that felt threatened by being thinner was probably screaming from within throughout her entire weight loss process. This unresolved, insecure part of her likely made her weight loss efforts more difficult and clearly made maintenance impossible. Her unresolved emotional blocks pulled her out of alignment and caused dissidence with her actions. Does this sound like a certain three-way you may know? This is similar to the sabotage trifecta of the fitness ménage à trois: needs being tolerated manifesting as coping mechanisms.

Maybe you've had a similar experience. Have you ever been absolutely committed to a diet? Think about a time when you were completely dedicated to losing weight. Come hell or high water, you did what was necessary in order to achieve your goal. You may have gone to parties or out to dinner and not once strayed from your diet. If tempted, you reminded yourself of your goal. Because you were so clear in knowing exactly what you should and should not eat and why, it was easier to resist the forbidden foods. As you persisted, you felt a boost of confidence by being able to stick to your commitment. Every day may not have been easy, but you stuck to it. All of your being was unified and strong: you were in alignment.

It wasn't until you decided that you were "off" your diet or thought you could cheat a little that things started falling apart. Usually, a dieter has a moment of indecision or cloudy thinking (misalignment) that turns into forsaking her goals and seeking retribution for the past two weeks, or months of deprivation. Justification, resentment, and hunger ban together unchecked to sabotage your intentions and drive you back onto the battlefield again!

Been there? Me too! Until you get your entire self into alignment, you'll continue to struggle. Alignment with the most authentic and powerful part of you will be your most glue-like type of inspiration. Not only will aligned goals inspire you, but being in a state of internal unity makes dissidence implausible: you're all on the same team! When your heart, mind, and spirit ban together, resolute action becomes easy and mutiny isn't an option.

How do you get to this aligned state? The first step is to access your authentic self—the real you or your highest self with her own set of values. These values are the bottom line for you; they are what your core self wants to express and experience in life. Authentic values are made up of what you hold most dear in the intangible realm, such as honesty, harmony, play, etc. In other words, alignment is getting your highest self in the driver's seat. Once you're clear about this sacred self, it's easy to set meaningful goals of similar theme and substance. Alignment is the unwavering power you seek—it is the glue of your self-care.

⌘ **Mental Fitness Exercise:** Recall when you have been in alignment with projects, undertakings, or goals in your recent or distant past. In which areas of your life do you have the least amount of struggle? When has your internal alignment worked for you? Make some notes on how you've used it to help yourself, or stay on track during tough times or important endeavors.

Go to www.loveyourselffit.com/inspiration for a downloadable version of this exercise.

CHAPTER 10

Higher Communication: Your Authentic Self and Guidance System

"In quietness are all things answered,
and is every problem quietly resolved."

A Course in Miracles

Fitness goals, career aspirations, or relationship repairs—whatever your goal—your authentic self is your truest guide; it's your inner compass.

Your authentic self is the essence of who you are emotionally, mentally, and spiritually. It's the part of you that dreams and aspires and begs to be expressed. It's the deepest truth of who you are without all your titles and roles. Your authentic self is your spirit embodied, and it can be expressed through mind, personality, and intuition.

Your authentic self can be called your Big-I. Your Big-I is bigger than you but completely whole within you. Your Big-I is you plus. It's your connection to everyone and everything that ever was or will be. Your

Big-I is synonymous with what the physicists call "the God particle". It's like the energetic building materials present in all things, throughout the universe and time. On the contrary, your ego or small, needier self is called your little-i.

When it comes to life direction, people tend to engage life like a sailing trip. Some steer their boats in a specific direction toward a desired destination; others figure it's easier to float with the current; and some just want to cruise around. Most of us never learn how to consult our inner compass for direction. Instead we head out on life's journey built on what we *think we should do* rather than what we deeply desire. We establish our course based on the opinions of others, psycho-emotional needs, or on the sea lane we think will offer the smoothest sailing, neglecting to listen to the authentic voice within. Thus, little-i thinking.

Not surprisingly, people tend to do the same thing with their fitness programs. They set out on a fitness plan based on what they think they *should do* to get themselves to where they think they *should be* without ever consulting their inner compass or body for direction. People tend to look outside of themselves for guidance, using parents, celebrities, or friends as role models for their choices. Founded in popular aesthetics or "expert" opinion, direction and motivation are grounded in the external input instead of inner wisdom. Little-i fitness, I call it.

Little-i thinking will lead you to seek quick fixes, external or fleeting pleasures, and immediate gratification. Your psycho-emotional needs will seem immeasurable, your thinking stressed, and you'll often feel unsatiated. You may feel resentment or a desire to rebel against the task, person, or project at hand. Conscious or not, internally something is out of congruence and becoming a source of dissidence between your intentions and your actions. This divided state may sound vaguely familiar. Diet, anyone?

Conversely, an authentic self is an empowered self. Therefore, seeking out and using your authentic self, your Big-I, as a guide is a means to building the self-care you've always wanted.

A Date—with Your Authentic Self

How can you meet your Big-I? Where is this authentic you hiding? It's not. It's already present. All you have to do is remove the interference blocking you from hearing it. Think of your authentic self as a radio station. You have to make an effort to tune into to that specific place to hear what's being broadcast from that station. If there's a lot of static around—noise, turbulent events, interactions, or thoughts—you'll be hard pressed to hear the broadcast. In other words, you can find your authentic self by quieting your mind and disconnecting from the external world, your roles, and what *The Crabby Angels Chronicles* author and spiritual boot camp leader Jacob Glass calls the "puppy-mind".

The puppy-mind is the hyper, bounce around, distractible mind-state in which many of us dwell much of the time. You might not realize how frequently your mind jumps subjects or rotates frantically on a specific line of thought. Seemingly unruly, your puppy-mind can appear to have ADHD, become obsessive, or generally be difficult to keep focused. Imagine your puppy-mind: yelping, whining, and barking loudly, shredding belongings, and crapping all over your (mental) house, leaving your authentic self as mere background noise. Your authentic self becomes comparable to the radio on low volume, left on in the other room.

Alignment with the authentic self means paper training your puppy-mind. It's actually a very simple practice; it only requires awareness and willingness. Initially, you must become aware of when your puppy is pooping on the sofa or floor (thoughts based in fear, anxiety, neediness, control, etc.) and then be willing to redirect him to the proverbial newspaper (thinking based in love, release, trust, etc.). The newspaper is where you want him to be soundly playing and doing his business. This newspaper for your puppy-mind is non-disruptive thinking, where the spastic, obsessive part of your mind can be sequestered or redirected, thus allowing you to tune in to your authentic radio station for guidance. If your puppy mind starts making a mess off the paper, dragging your mind through negative thoughts or fears, you don't beat him, scream, or start obsessing about what a horrible, incapable dog he is. You gently and clearly bring him back to the newspaper, calm and clear. When your thinking is obsessive or becomes fractious, you bring it back to where you want it to be. It's a simple and conscious effort to redirect your thoughts. Instead of allowing your mind to run amuck and think whatever, whenever it wants, or dive into horror stories about your fatness or oldness, you bring it back to where you want it to be. Your first line to authenticity then is to deliberately choose your line of thought; focus your mind and gently correct when necessary.

Imagine you're driving home from work replaying a heated conversation you had with a coworker and repetitively continue to chastise yourself for saying the wrong thing. You think of all of the things you should have said instead of what you did say. This leads into thoughts about how inept you are at communicating with others or how poorly you communicate with your family, and so on. You're essentially beating your puppy-mind with the newspaper instead of directing him to it! Instead, choose to calmly bring your cute little thoughts to the newspaper by shifting your thinking to the opposite line of thought—in this case to what you said well today. Maybe you gave someone a compliment on appearance or handled an ethical violation with incredible tact...bring your thoughts to those. Where do you want your puppy? What do you want to be thinking? Do you want to swim in the pool of your ineptitude or dive into your capabilities? Would you teach your child with verbal abuse or direct him to the appropriate behavior? Behaviorists, teachers, and animal trainers all know the most effective forms of training aren't those brought by punishment. Rather it's to focus on the behavior you do want to establish and encourage that.

So must you do so with your mind: redirect your thoughts, praise what's positive, repeat. Redirect, praise, repeat seeds the energy of gratitude.

Redirection is helpful and your most formidable path to authentic self—by calming your puppy-mind. When you calm the puppy-mind, you have an opportunity to awaken your authentic self via Big-I time. This sacred or Big-I time is an opportunity for divine communication, or a date with your spirit. You set aside Big-I time to recharge your soul-u-lar battery. Your attention is turned inward, away from demands and to-do lists, away from noise and external stimuli. You gather your energy and attention and focus it inward. You become quiet and centered. Big-I time is the ultimate state of being-ness, where you allow yourself to be divinely guided, connecting with your most powerful self and Big-I thinking.

This sacred time can take many different forms, and you aren't limited to one. It may or may not involve a religious belief. It could be a part of connecting with a higher power or simply quieting the mind. Meditation is an ideal practice of Big-I or sacred time. You can begin your meditation with a question in mind and allow your highest self to answer. For some people prayer, breath work, or chanting are sacred practices. For others, religious ceremony or scripture may fulfill the order. I do encourage you to do less cerebral practices; try one that allows conscious functioning of the ego to take a backseat. The key characteristic is that this time quiets the puppy-mind and allows for a deeper connection with spirit, with your authentic or Big-I.

Journaling or writing can be therapeutic and a good focusing exercise. It also provides a good lead-in to sacred time. For some, body movement is the gate. Tai Chi, Qigong, and yoga are all centering physical practices. Sacred music—or music that resonates with your spirit—is a wonderful means of bringing your mind to be calm and centered. Breathing techniques are also a calming physical and mental tool.

The paths of Big-I time are varied, but its effects are consistent: a quiet, centered mind. The results are calmness, clarity, and a peaceful, recharged energy. The health benefits of practices such as meditation are well documented and growing. Stress reduction, decreased depression and anxiety, blood pressure and hormone regulation are but a few of the rewards you'll reap as a regular meditator. The action of quieting the mind shifts your energy so your vibration becomes calm and centered too. This calm peacefulness enters the realm of what Catherine Ponder calls Divine Love in her book *The Prospering Power of Love.* Sacred time is the most important part of your self-care practice. I'm not sure all trainers or doctors would agree, but state of mind is the most dominant factor in an individual's overall wellbeing.

Schedule sacred time as you would any other appointment. I highly recommend a morning practice for your Big-I or sacred time. Setting aside sacred time and space for your authentic self first thing in the morning collects the puppy-mind and makes it sit and stay. This doesn't mean it won't wander off during the day, but it starts your mind in the ideal state before you go out into the world to interact with your job, your family, or relationships. It's self-care of the highest kind.

If you don't know how to meditate or practice deep breathing, don't worry. Plenty of instruction is available free of charge online or at your local library. Again, tap the available resources, explore and experiment, and find out what awakens your spirit.

⌘ **Mental Fitness Exercise:** What do you know about your authentic self? Do you have any inklings about what your most sacred, spiritual self dreams of or desires? If your authentic self can be found in the silencing of your puppy-mind, how will you quiet yourself? Write at least two ways you will spend your Big-I time or sacred-self dates.

⌘ **Mental Fitness Exercise:** Begin a morning practice of Big-I time. It can be just five minutes of meditation or quiet, sacred time. Use the ideas in this book to start your practice. This is the most important piece of your self-care practice, so don't blow this one off!

⌘ **Mental Fitness Exercise:** Can you picture your puppy-mind? What kind of a puppy is it? Does he/she have a name? And do you have any techniques or ideas about calming, or redirecting him/her? If you have none, invent some. Know what to do to redirect your puppy-mind.

Go to www.loveyourselffit.com/inspiration for a downloadable version of these exercises.

CHAPTER 11

Defining Your Body-Mind Relationship: Using Values to Set Meaningful Goals

*"What is false in the science of facts may be
true in the science of values."*

George Santayana

Pretend for a moment you're at a funeral. You're a mouse in the corner and you hear a woman eulogizing her best friend. "Bianca was such a gorgeous woman. She was a beautiful lady. Did you ever see her in a bikini? My God! She looked fabulous! She had a perfect butt and the flattest stomach. She worked on her body constantly, running every day, and she spent two or three hours at the gym. And boy-oh-boy, were those surgeries worth every penny!"

She goes on. "Bianca always enjoyed the best: she had a great house, nice cars, and beautiful clothing. Her taste was impeccable. She only wore the latest, never anything last season. There wasn't a day or night she didn't look perfect. Although, sometimes she'd get a little cranky from the 800 calorie-a-day diets and was regularly laid up from all the voluntary procedures, her dog Atkins and I will always remember her fondly."

It may sound a bit silly, but is this the type of eulogy you'd want delivered at your funeral? Who was Bianca? Was anything said about the real Bianca—as a person? Her experiences? Her contributions? Her relations with anyone (but herself)? And yet, ask yourself how much time you spend thinking about those exact same things in her eulogy: your appearance, clothing, home, or car? How often do you worry, complain, lament, feel guilty about, or plot to change your looks? How often do you think about your weight, food, dieting, or what you *should* be eating? Do you think about it when you go to the refrigerator or the closet, or on a night out, or to work or school? How often do you cringe at your photograph? How often do you avoid something you would really love to do because of your weight or appearance?

Thinking about the bigger picture of your life and the experiences, people, and activities you value most is incredibly beneficial. You might think a eulogy is morbid or scary, but it's simply a tool for identifying your authentic values. Consider what you really want in the whole of your life, and compare this to how you're currently spending your time, energy, and money. Would anyone, close enough to you to deliver your eulogy, talk about the size or shape of your ass? (Assuming you're not J-Lo, of course.) Or how you looked in a bikini in 2014? Perhaps your beloved friend would discuss those dynamite shoes you wore that one night to that one party… remember those? Of course not! Because some of what you give your life, money, energy, and brain to is irrelevant, pretty much a waste of your time, and not what people remember about you. I like cute shoes too—it's part of the female genome—but you may not realize how much of your time and energy you're spending on elements that aren't aligned with your highest values.

Imagine your life as a bag of coins, and each day's thoughts, feelings, desires, actions, and language (all forms of energy!) are coins spent from that bag. Are you *spending your life* on Big-I stuff or little-i stuff? Do you limit your thoughts or actions, because in one way or another you're not "good enough"? Do you believe plastic surgery or reaching your ideal weight will make you happy or change your experience? If reaching your goal weight were a happy pill, would you ever regain lost weight? Would anyone?

Eventually the day of your funeral will come and your life will have served some purpose, reflected some value, or embraced some element or passion that was most important to you. Your life is an experience and a statement. In fact, you're making a statement with your life right now and will continue to do so every minute of every day either by directed intention or by passive choice.

Now, take a moment and think about what you *would* want said about you and about your life. If people will remember how they felt in your presence, what would you like them to recall? How do you want to feel in the presence of others? What are the most relevant things for you to contribute and experience? Reflect on what's most important to *you* in your daily routine: joy, laughter, loving relationships, security? Write your ideal eulogy.

You can use this eulogy to define the essence of your values. Using your eulogy, make a list of the possessions and experiences you want most in your lifetime or everydays. Then, next to each item or experience write the essence of it. In other words, next to "my own business" I would write "freedom, power, or meaningful contribution". Perhaps the essence of having "a beautiful home" would be living in a serene environment or sanctuary. These essence elements are your authentic values. Your essence elements are what you desire most and that which inspires you to take action. These are the values that get you out of bed in the morning and explain your choice in mates. They're the essence, content, or truth of what's most important to you. The business and house are the form, outcome, or what I call the middleman which you believe will give you the essence of what you seek. You may think the perfect body will give confidence, money will assure security, or a baby will bring love. Then you find out the confidence is conditional, the money brings more fear than security, and the baby becomes a teenager and "hates" you for quite a while. Middlemen are alluring but they usually make you a long-term custodian of a short term fix. Often we mistakenly seek the middleman of form thinking it will bring us the experience or essence of what we want.

You can easily mistake the middleman for the essence, so it's important for you to know the difference. Compare what you're spending your time, thoughts, and energy on every day and ask yourself: am I in alignment with my Big-I values or am I focusing on acquisition of form and hoping the middleman will deliver? Look for discrepancies and synergistic elements. In which ways are you living in harmony with your authentic values, and where do you need to redirect, praise, repeat?

I would guess that a tight ass and chiseled abs are not on your authentic values list. I would even go so far as to say: *Your soul don't give a squirt of piss about your body fat percentage!* (It reads better if you say it with a southern drawl.) Fitness and health simply usher into your life time and ease: more time on the planet and the ease of good function. They allow your spirit the time to express its beauty and love. A healthy body is a catalyst to enjoying life; it's easier to thrive with a fit, strong body.

Using authentic values simply hooks you into your internal motivators, a.k.a. aligned inspiration. These values will help you most if you refresh or remind your mind daily. Because the world we live in is so full of information, ideas, and sparkly things (think "Squirrel!"), you have to input daily the concepts that you want to keep front and center. Anything from notes on your mirror, or pictures that stir up a feeling or thought, to your phone set to send you memos that remind you of your authentic values will work. Alignment starts with identifying your inspiration (authentic values) but sticks with fresh, daily doses.

Just as a marriage will flourish when both partners are in sync, so shall this budding relationship of your body-mind fitness blossom when all of you is in sync, focused on the same direction, and using your authentic values to make meaningful self-care goals.

⌘ **Mental Fitness Exercise:** Write your eulogy and use it to pull out the essence elements you really want to create an authentic values list. You'll use these authentic values to set meaningful self-care goals that resonate with your authentic self and inspire you from within.

⌘ **Mental Fitness Exercise:** Make note of the thoughts or beliefs you've established that have attached your physical appearance with your internal experience. For example, you want your body to be _____ so you experience the sense of _____. Question those. Are they based in Big-I love, or little-i neediness or fear? And would you want your spouse or friend saying the same thing to you: "I want your body to be thin so I experience a sense of pride (being with you)." How does that feel to you?

⌘ **Mental Fitness Exercise:** Once you're familiar with some of your authentic values, choose which forms of refreshment will be most helpful to you: pictures, recordings, videos, quotes, sayings, poems, etc. Where or how will you refresh? Will you hang sayings on your bathroom mirror or steering wheel, listen to a recording on your way to work, or make a picture your phone background? Begin a practice of refreshing your authentic values.

🖱 Go to www.loveyourselffit.com/inspiration for a downloadable version of these exercises.

Setting Meaningful Goals

When I first begin working with a new client, I ask her to list her fitness goals. Interestingly, what usually happens over the course of coaching is that we find these goals to be unauthentic. Usually they're extrinsic or based on input and images from outside of her. If pursued, these extrinsic goals will lead her down the same effortful paths she has previously taken. She must run her goals through the authentic filter.

It's tempting to base your fitness goals on what you think you *should* look like. It's not uncommon to measure yourself against the numbers touted by a chart, a publication, an expert, or your high school or pre-baby cognitive weight records, or the clothing corpses from any of these eras—still hanging in your closet. I call these "shouldy" goals. (Phonic pun intended!) Shouldy goals, those born of the ego, are usually extrinsic and therefore ineffective.

Shouldy, extrinsic goals are weak and unhelpful, and unfortunately aesthetic goals are just plain shouldy. You may have started a fitness program with your goals and ambition firmly grounded in a "look fabulous" fantasy. However, if being beautiful were a strong enough motivator, you wouldn't be struggling with fitness at all. Your vanity would take care of your eating issues and exercise resistance for you! You would have long ago reached your goals and have little trouble maintaining them. Though you may share your society's obsession with beauty, it's not an *authentic value* for you. (This means you're super deep. As in writing poetry and wearing little-square-shaped-sunglasses-indoors deep. Seriously, your values are deeper and that's a good thing.) Therefore, you need more than the extrinsic, bimbo-riffic oriented goal to alter your everyday behavior.

When you're alone at night with a craving for chocolate ice cream or potato chips, the notion of looking thinner in two weeks isn't going to rescue you from your pantry tonight. There's a stronger motivator at work within you, pulling you in a different direction. Beauty as a future destination doesn't stand up to your unanswered psycho-emotional needs or food-horniness in the present. The desire to be thin is likely not an intrinsic goal or a large enough part of who you are authentically to be a strong enough motivator on its own. Aesthetics are a great motivator for some people, but not all of us. If it were a key motivator for you, you'd think of your bikini and walk away from the chips and ice cream!

If aesthetic goals haven't sustained your commitment to self-care yet, they probably won't start working for you now! Let's be honest: haven't you been trying to do this with the goal of "weigh 120 pounds" or "wear a size 6" forever? How's that working? What's the definition of insanity again? If you're afraid to release your grip on making a physical outcome goal, you may have some resistance or fear that you're unaware of operating in the background. Investigation is your friend.

If your goals are not from you, don't resonate with you, and won't fit into your life, they won't be maintainable. Like choosing a bra off the rack that's marked "one size fits all", a self-care practice that doesn't fit you won't work for long. Something that originated from outside of you that doesn't mesh with your body, values, schedule, or tastes isn't going to be something you can put on every day and be happy and content with. You want to create a self-care program that fits you like a custom-tailored suit. You'll love it, or at least like it, and feel great "wearing it" every day. When a goal is in alignment with who you are, it will be inspiring, interesting, and fun. It will feel like that new outfit that you can't wait to wear.

Meaningful goals are the type of goal I encourage you to set. Making a meaningful goal is a commitment to a behavior with the process, experience, or mindset as the priority. Authentic values work well in conjunction with meaningful goals, because they're both rooted in your conscious experience.

Use your authentic values to make meaningful goals. If you listed an authentic value of "freedom" or "power", an example of a meaningful goal might include exercises that make you feel powerful like strength training or movement that enables the feeling of freedom like trail running. You can also use your authentic values as a catalyst for self-care. If your authentic values include "loving relationships with grandchildren", your meaningful goals may be directed toward actualizing more time with or focused energy on your grandchildren. These goals could be something like "Walk for 20 minutes four times a week" which is directly connected to a values-based outcome goal of "keeping up with Rebecca and Shawn at the zoo".

Meaningful goals generally are a practice you prioritize and commit to, regardless of outcome or results. The same way you would make a goal with your relationship: a daily hug or "I love you", talking about finances once a month, or making him a nice meal on Fridays, meaningful goals are about your daily practice and experience. Exercising three days a week, using kind words with yourself in the bathroom mirror, or redirecting your puppy-mind when it starts tearing up your mental living room are all examples of meaningful self-care goals. You can also make them simple baby steps that have little or nothing to do with your authentic values. For instance, taking your vitamins after lunch or eating a green vegetable twice a day is a small and simple meaningful goal. Conversely, an outcome goal is one based on results, such as a goal of weighing 120 pounds. If you focus on an outcome, make sure it's an energy or experience you desire, like finishing the mud-run, feeling strong at the gym or sexy in that black dress, and not a numerical measurement.

Meaningful goals are a prerequisite to outcome goals. You can try to reach an outcome goal without learning the mindset and behaviors that will maintain that outcome—but you won't retain the results. After all, meaningful goals are the meat. They're the reality of fitness: sustaining healthy behaviors daily. Moreover, when you get "there" (to your desired outcome goal), what's waiting for you is the same thing you've done all along…the daily practice! Funny how that works. Creating meaningful goals are the next big step in making your mind-body connection and relationship.

"What about the numbers, charts, experts, and SMART goals?" you ask. This may sound like sacrilege for a fitness trainer to say, but setting an outcome goal based on numbers is like trying to stay in a miserable marriage just so you can say, "We've been married for fifteen years." You want to get that crystal watch badly, don't you honey?

Numbers and dates are things to celebrate along the way, not the purpose of being together.

Establishing a marriage with the objective of being together for twenty-three years is ridiculous. It's just as ridiculous as starting a fitness practice with the goal of achieving some random number on the scale or calipers. Numbers and weight loss are things to celebrate along the way, not the object of your self-care! Your body's health, weight, strength, and body fat percentage are variable, changing throughout the years you're alive. Additionally, an ideal set of numbers, sizes, and measurements randomly contrived for the masses is poppycock. (For those of you familiar with *Fancy Nancy,* poppycock is a fancy word for bullshit.)

Setting a goal of reaching the twenty-three year mark in a marriage is a dumb SMART goal. It's Specific, Measurable, Attainable, Relevant, and Time-bound, but will it ever work to make a long, happy marriage? No. SMART goals are dumb when it comes to marriage and self-care, because they're both relationships in which you want the same experience: a pleasant, loving—even joyful—process you can live with every day. You want them both to last a long time and be easy to maintain. Numbers are a measurement of the ego, not your highest self, and they do little to improve a relationship. Relationships are fed by a daily practice and joyful experiences. Numerical outcome goals negate the everyday experience which, in turn, destroys longevity.

If you don't want to make meaningful goals, write a fitness mission statement instead. A mission statement clarifies the direction and intent of a body or organization. It's a guide, a shared goal, and an agreed way of operating. You can create a fitness statement for your self-care practice.

This can be fun, because you get to suspend your current reality and play with what you want for yourself. Yes, I said fun! Suspend reality and your negative past experiences. Pretend you can have your exercise and eating any way you want it to be. How would it be? If you could choose the thoughts and feelings you would have going to the gym, what would they be? Describe them. When you sit down for a meal, what do you want to be thinking about the food in front of you? Would you feel the sensations more clearly in your body? Write it all down. Let yourself go with a moment of fantasy, and connect to what you really want for yourself in your daily life. Focus on how you want your everyday experience to be instead of fixating on a number-based outcome. Do you want to unconditionally love your body and smile when you look at yourself in the mirror (instead of fight with the bitch)? Do you want to listen perfectly to your body's messages when it comes to food? Do you want to look forward to exercising? Suspend your can'ts and doubts long enough to jot down some direction. (Ask yourself the same questions to make your goals.)

Having a fitness statement, an ideal in mind, really helped me to change my relationship to food. When it came to eating, I felt like a prisoner of an immortal habit. I hated this feeling. I tried a thousand different ways to deal with my problem without success. What I didn't realize all along was that my focus was misplaced.

Though my true desire was to be free of using food as a coping mechanism, I never focused on resolving my coping mechanism or healing my emotional drivers as a goal. Instead, my goal had always been to lose weight, weigh a certain amount, or control my eating. I was always trying to manipulate my eating and my body to make my body skinny. The goal of having a healthy perception of food or to listen to my body never crossed my mind. I thought if I found a way to get skinny (outcome) and have control over food (outcome), I would be free (essence) of my eating addiction and live happily ever after (essence). I was wrong. Focusing on getting skinny only made me crazier about food and my body fatter. Focus expands.

Though I wanted to be thin, it wasn't until I ultimately grasped that what I *really* wanted was to be free of eating as a coping mechanism. This is when I started to shift. When I focused on the content of what I really wanted, I realized my ideal was to be able to eat whatever and whenever, without rules or measuring cups. I wanted to have a healthy, natural relationship to food and listen to my body. I wanted to be able to eat any kind of food and stop when or before I was full. I didn't want to have food "issues" anymore; I wanted to be free! And of course I wanted to be leaner, but I wanted my body weight to balance itself in its natural range. I didn't want to fight the war any longer.

As if light rays shone down from the sky, it dawned on me: what if I could actually be free? What if I could be free to enjoy food *and* listen to my body? The concept was foreign, yet very inspiring to me. I started to consider this ideal an actual possibility and made it my goal. I began focusing on "being free" instead of "getting skinny". I wrote my ideal on a piece of paper and held it in my mind as often as I could. I soon found myself reflexively being led to the necessary work to achieve a healthy way of being with food, dealing with what drove me to use food as a coping mechanism, and learning to listen to my body.

Without shifting my focus to the authentic value (freedom) and holding the "being free" ideal in my mind as a reality, I'm not sure I could have changed my eating behaviors. My energy had been focused on controlling food and trying to manipulate my body to be skinny, a.k.a. resisting fat and fixating on the middleman or form. In truth, all this did was make "fat" fill my consciousness. I was always thinking, "I want to lose weight. I'm fat", but the energy in my mind and body was simply focused on "FAT" and "WEIGHT" and "LOSS". When I shifted my focus to "A healthy relationship with food" and "I easily listen to my body", the energy in my mind and body was now "HEALTHY" and "RELATIONSHIP" and "LISTEN". I believed my ideal was possible, and my whole being shifted to match. My behavior soon followed, and eventually my ideal grew to reality. Remember, this is all about your mental and emotional energy and focus! Your focus determines your energy and your energy creates your experience and shapes your outcome.

This concept of focusing your mind on an ideal is not new. It's actually quite ancient! Philosophy, religion, psychology, even pop-culture all echo this principle. Remember "Feel the force, Luke" from the movie *Star Wars?* What you focus on expands. Resistance only makes what you're pushing against push back. Focus on the essence or content of what you want to experience every day in terms of self-care and make that your goal. The fitness statement or written goal is an official statement and a reminder for you.

⌘ **Mental Fitness Exercise:** Question yourself about your goals. Ask and answer: what am I afraid will happen if I let go of my aesthetics-based outcome goal(s)? And then what? Repeat "And then what?" until you get down to that place or statement that scares you a little bit or feels uncomfortable. This is the source of resistance to flowing with your meaningful goals and finding your true inspiration. This is an issue where you can use the CORE, or work with a skilled coach or therapist.

⌘ **Mental Fitness Exercise:** Bail the extrinsic, shouldy goals you would normally set for your body and fitness and go for content rich, meaningful goals. Use your authentic values (the essence elements of your eulogy) to help you outline some inspirational goals. Avoid numbers and the dumb SMART idea.

⌘ **Mental Fitness Exercise:** Answer the fitness mission statement questions in the body of this chapter. Ask yourself: How will I know when I'm practicing great self-care? How will I feel? What will I do and how often? What will I think about my body, exercise, food, weight, etc.?

Go to www.loveyourselffit.com/inspiration for a downloadable version of these exercises.

SECTION IV

Building a Body-Loving Relationship

CHAPTER 12

Falling in Love with You: Wrapping Up the Beauty Box

"Love is not something you look for...
love is something you become."

Alina Villasante

Remember that mean, old boyfriend from Chapter 3? The flesh-pinching, comparison-making loser you put up with in your dream didn't help you succeed, feel good about yourself, or keep your commitments. Time to break up!

Fitness, beauty, or weight loss achieved with a loveless state of mind is not self-care, not real self-esteem; it's conditional and disrespectful. Deluding yourself into believing that "looking good" will end your loveless relationship or that you can appease the abuser within by becoming more attractive is a fool's errand. The abuser will arise as soon as you gain a pound, incur a scar, discover a wrinkle, lose or grow hair, or have a birthday. Hating your body in order to love it is an illogical and ineffective platform for self-care.

Self-care can't be cruel, judgmental, or unloving. Loveless-ness begets the same. If your fitness strategy is based in judgment or cruelty to the body, it's not fitness or self-care; it's ego-care or aesthetic building. Like a loving LTR, lasting self-care comes from love, acceptance, and understanding. It has to be something positive if you expect to feel good maintaining it.

Because the Loveless Marriage comes from valuing beauty over well-being, your first step in building a loving relationship with yourself is to investigate beauty as a cultural and personal value and decide where it belongs in your reality.

The Beauty Box

We all want to be beautiful. Beauty is associated with power, preference, value, and love, especially for women. Beauty has long been the feminine form of currency in many cultures. Today, beauty has become a cultural mindset: we strive for it, pay just about any sum to have it, and go to the most extreme lengths to get it.

The way we think about beauty is so embedded in our social norms that we've come to unconsciously embrace beliefs that are detrimental to our wellbeing. The loveless relationship we've built with our bodies is often a result of, and perpetuated by, this limited mind-state I call the beauty box.

Throughout my lifetime I've noticed an unconscious loyalty amongst women, in differing degrees, to the beauty box. Women regularly commune and rehash the same mantras about beautification procedures, weight loss efforts, and anti-aging treatments, coupled with the latest weaponry for this ongoing war we're fighting. We read books and magazines about achieving beauty, think about it, emotionally belabor it, and invest a significant amount of money and time into it. Women watch the shows, buy the products, pay for the procedures, do the diets, pop the pills, and lament our own shortcomings ad nauseam. We buy into society's standards of beauty, a.k.a. the beauty box, and accept this beauty-centric lifestyle as a normal part of being a woman.

There's an unspoken rule if you're female: you had better look as good as you can for as long as you can. Buy into the beauty box or pay the social consequences, baby! If you don't, you'll be considered asexual, lazy, unhealthy, unhappy, unsuccessful, and unattractive. Not embracing beauty is a form of rejection of the norms of society and the feminine role. Consider the way women talk about other women. "Rebecca would be such a pretty girl if she just lost some weight." Or "It's such a pity; she's really let herself go!" If you meet a new woman at a party or watch celebrities at award shows, don't you assess them based on their looks? Beauty box judgment is a habit. Women regularly hold women to the standards we've grown accustomed to holding all females: the beauty box.

When your best friend is dating a loser, you know it. You think to yourself, "She found an asshole who treats her like dog crap and she won't leave him." You know there are a thousand better men out there for her, but she can't see this, because she's so wrapped up in this relationship. The same is true with the beauty box. Women are so wrapped up in our beliefs and pursuits of beauty that we can't see how lame it is. There are a thousand better ways to treat all the female bodies around us—celebrity, neighbor, and self—than to continuously measure them against the beauty box.

For most of us, our cultural beauty obsession feeds a negative body image. We've all heard the stats on female body image and underage girls' weight obsession. The trouble, when it comes to negative body image and self-care, is that the former reduces the later. The more active your contempt for something or someone, the worse you treat it or them. Thus the Loveless Marriage is conceived.

You may think idolizing the beauty box helps you keep your eating under control or motivates you to exercise. But *does it really?* If you were honest with yourself, wouldn't it feel more like someone outside of you trying to manipulate you with fear of rejection or loss of love? Have a friend say to you the things you say to yourself about beauty, weight, and having to look good and then decide if those words are helpful.

Eye of the Beholder

What if you find Prince Charming, but he isn't exactly great looking? He has all the qualities you want in a mate, and you're extremely attracted to him, but he's not traditionally handsome. He's smart, kind, chivalrous, great in bed, tall, funny, well spoken, very sexy, and has a great career; he has it all except that he's not cute. Do you throw him back because he isn't beautiful? Briefly think about what you want in a partner and from a relationship. Is your mate's appearance as vital as a deep connection or his communication skills? Can a pretty smile beat generosity or ambition? Would your passion for him be dwarfed by his external packaging? In other words, would you pick the box with the pretty packaging over the one with the really good stuff inside? And if you would choose the pretty one, what will you do as time passes? Even the most gorgeous wrapping paper and ribbon fades and withers in time.

Think about physical beauty for a moment. Where does it fit into your life? How important is being beautiful? Is it crucial to a fulfilling and happy life for you? Have you considered how big a part of your life "looking good naked" is each day?

How much of your day do you need to look good naked? Two percent of your day, if you looked at or had another person look at your naked body, for thirty minutes a day, every day. Keep in mind that's if you want to invest thirty minutes per day on looking at yourself naked in the mirror! It may also be important to look good naked the three days a decade you have sex, with the lights on or during daylight, or perhaps when you go to the beach in a very, very skimpy bikini. That's it. Compare this two percent of actual time to the amount of energy, thought, and kvetch-time you give it. Could it be this "looking good naked" thing is slightly overrated as a meaningful component of your life?

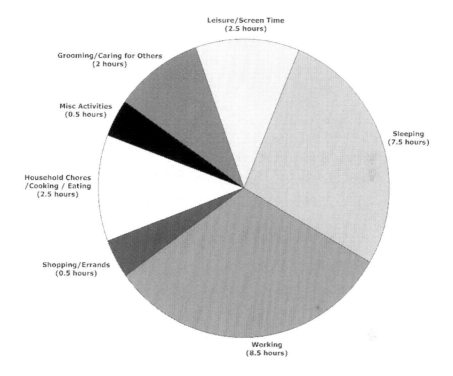

Leisure/Screen Time
(2.5 hours)

Grooming/Caring for Others
(2 hours)

Misc Activities
(0.5 hours)

Sleeping
(7.5 hours)

Household Chores
/Cooking / Eating
(2.5 hours)

Shopping/Errands
(0.5 hours)

Working
(8.5 hours)

Total= 24.0 hours

NOTE: Graphic inspired by chart from the Bureau of Labor Statistics, American Time Use Survey

If you consider all that you long to experience and express in your life, physical beauty probably pales in comparison. Reflect on your authentic values and eulogy. Consult your wisest self. What do you want to contribute to the human race? Nice abs? Great tits? Will you strive to leave your family the legacy of a wrinkle-free face or something greater? Which would you prefer: "Aunt Beth had amazing skin" or "Aunt Beth founded the Lymphoma Research Institute, which paved the way for many blood-related cancer treatments"? Think about the contribution you could make to the world via time, money, or energy with what you now (or may be planning to) spend on personal beautification.

I'm not trying to throw a guilt dart at you if you want to buy cute shoes or get a facelift. We're all enriched by beauty, including the beauty of outward appearances. Yet, so many women believe and behave as if beauty is our *greatest* contribution to society or the most valuable part of our selves. It's not. But we keep that myth alive for ourselves and for the little girls growing up around us, with our beautification investments of time, money and energy.

Most people want to look their best, as do I, and there's nothing wrong with this. The problem arises when beauty is held at a higher priority than mind, heart, knowledge, health or wellbeing, spirit, expression, or relationships. When our little girls are more concerned about being fat at age seven than learning to read or communicate effectively, or gyrating four-year-olds on stage get an hour of primetime television with more make-up than Tammy Faye, some part of you must be alarmed. (Please tell me you're alarmed.) This distortion in perspective occurs when we lose grasp of where beauty lies in the whole of our lives, and we end up making it more important than the things that really matter. An ill state of mind, depression, obsession, or despondence about the shape or size of your body, because it isn't fitting into the current beauty box is exactly this distortion in perspective and an all-too-common occurrence among females of all ages.

I'm not anti-cosmetic. In fact, I appreciate and use beauty enhancers. I have had plastic surgery (granted, it was for a medical reason), but I was and continue to be grateful to professionals who specialize in those procedures. They have amazing skills, help so many people, and continue to create less invasive and health-risking procedures. Yet, beauty is a matter of balance and perspective. When health and beauty are held in perspective, cosmetics hurt no one.

This begs the question of investment. Beauty is alluring, but is it a good investment? No. In fact, it's a poor investment of resources. If we were to analyze the financial investment Americans make in the name of beauty, based on what we spend for dieting, cosmetics, and plastic surgery, we would find it's enough to feed a small country. According to recent reports and estimates, we spend almost one hundred billion dollars annually trying to be pretty.[7,8,9] That's a lot of dog shelters! What about the dividends? Ask a financial advisor about an investment costing you thousands of dollars a year that's not liquid, not tax deductible, and non-transferable. While becoming more costly to maintain each year, this investment yields high margins for its retailers but will never produce a profit for you or your heirs. Hmmm, I wonder what your financial advisor would say.

Aesthetic goals are a good example of the middleman or form over essence. It's feeling attractive, magnetic, sexy, alluring, powerful, adored, or treasured that make up what we truly desire, and these belong to anyone who will claim them. Embrace, embody and believe, and "beauty" will be yours. You don't actually have to look beautiful to attract, or feel loved, valued, or powerful. I'm sure you've known at least one person in your lifetime who wasn't the most physically gorgeous creature on the planet but who was extremely attractive and had no problem attracting mates or exuding self-confidence.

I remember a girl from high school who was "not much to look at". She was quite hard featured and not a looker, if you catch my meaning. Yet she always had an adorable boyfriend. They were good looking, sweet, private school kind of chaps. She pulled them in like ants at a picnic. (And she wasn't doing or wearing anything the rest of us weren't!) It was something about the way she carried herself that was intoxicating to these guys.

Putting beauty in perspective amongst your personal values will allow you to create a loving relationship with your body and positively affect your self-care. And this is the next step in creating a loving relationship with yourself. To be mentally fit and live in our culture with self-love, I chose to put beauty into perspective for myself. I'm not on this planet to be a model or a beauty queen. I know that my greatest strength doesn't lie in my looks; nor do my looks make up my greatest contribution to society. There are other aspects of me that are much more worthwhile than the features of my face, the definition in my arms, or the shape of my butt. This doesn't mean I don't try to look my best, appreciate my own beauty, or that if I look beautiful I'm a bad person. Beauty is not bad; beauty is neutral. It's an obsession with beauty that can be harmful.

Only you can decide what's most important to you and where beauty sits amongst your values. You're the only one able to determine if it's absolutely necessary in order for you to experience love. Is beauty a standard you're willing to set in all your relationships? In other words, will you require all those you love to be beautiful, young, or thin? If not, then why would you require it of yourself? Do your relationships with good looking people differ in terms of quality? Are they better or more fulfilling? If you set a standard of beauty for all the people in your life, good luck. (And lose my number please!)

If beauty is contributing to your self-care and behavior, then keep it in your tool box. Otherwise, decide to change your beliefs about beauty. Make your health, intelligence, spirituality, career success, happiness, or relationships more important. Find a way to make beauty the frosting on your cake of life, instead of the cake itself.

Prioritizing a healthy, balanced lifestyle will lead you to longevity, fitness, and your best weight. You can't say the same about choosing beauty or weight loss as your self-care focus. Making beauty your priority can lead you to unhealthy results like eating disorders, yo-yo dieting, pill popping, repetitive surgeries, disease, stress, and injuries. Health will always serve you and create beauty, while beauty merely serves itself.

⌘ **Mental Fitness Exercise:** Write down the statements you regularly make about yourself and your body in regards to your appearance. You don't have to disclose intent, but have a friend or mate read them aloud to you "in character". How do those statements feel when someone else says them to you? Do you feel inspired, hurt, delighted, or angry? Would those statements be ones you would use to inspire a child or friend? If a twelve year-old girl would cry or say "Whatever!" you need to get rid of them. You want keepers that conjure positive effects or feel inspiring.

⌘ **Mental Fitness Exercise:** Investigate your beliefs about beauty. Rank beauty among your authentic values. Decide where it sits compared to wellbeing and write an affirmative statement about your choice.

⌘ **Mental Fitness Exercise:** How can you make beauty the icing on your life cake instead of the cake itself? In the face of our beauty-obsessed culture, how will you keep it in perspective?

Go to www.loveyourselffit.com/inspiration for a downloadable version of these exercises.

CHAPTER 13

Opening to Love:
New Lenses

"We come to love not by finding a perfect person,
but by learning to see an imperfect person perfectly."

Sam Keen

After you turned four, have you ever loved your body and thought it was *absolutely* perfect as it is? Perhaps there were times when you've felt better about your looks, but do you remember a time when you said, "Okay, this is it, I'm there!"? If so, how long did your approval last? Was the acceptance you had genuine or was it conditionally based on maintaining that state?

In fact, most of us view ourselves and our bodies through distorted lenses. We constantly tell ourselves we need to look better: we're not good enough, thin enough, or young enough. Most people never feel anywhere near perfect, no matter how great their appearance. Even the world's top models think their looks can be improved. Their bodies may seem perfect to others, but not in their own perceptions.

There may have been a time in your life, five, ten, or forty pounds or years ago, that you look back upon now with envy. In retrospect, you wish you were still that weight or age. Yet, if you recall the mind-state you had then, you probably weren't satisfied with your body. You may have thought you could still be a little thinner, taller, or better looking in one way or another. You weren't present in the beauty and body you had. You're probably still not present in the beauty in which you sit right now. You've likely always viewed yourself through the eyes of your littlest self, your ego. But the ego is never satisfied. When it comes to the ego's perspective, there's always better or more to be achieved.

One's external reality doesn't always match one's internal perception, as disorders like body dysmorphic disorder and anorexia demonstrate. Your own perceptions of your body throughout the years may point to the same idea as well. How many different celebrities can you think of who have mildly (or severely) mutated themselves out of a skewed self-perception? I can think of a couple! You're wearing judgment-colored glasses and will never truly love your body until you change the prescription.

It doesn't matter how you actually look, it's what you believe about how you look that determines your level of body satisfaction.

Changing your body image, and hence your level of body satisfaction, means changing the lenses through which you view your body. Your current goggles are distorted; they're colored with judgment and shaped by mass media. Your optical prescription has been filled by an optometrist who wants you to always see yourself as flawed so he can continue to sell you products, services, and procedures to "fix" yourself. This optometrist will never offer you love-colored glasses to nurture your body, for to do so would put him out of business. You must replace your prescription with love-colored lenses if you want to love your body, and this is your next step to establishing a love-based relationship.

If your positive self-image is based on looking good, don't kid yourself into thinking that you've established genuine self-love. This is a conditional love relationship with your body. This pseudo self-love is based on maintaining your appearance. Like the woman who marries the man for his money, or the friend who's only friendly when you're buying, your love or self-image is based on a superficial foundation. You've set yourself up for a lifetime of conditional confidence, dependent esteem, and so-called self-love, all based on your appearance.

So what's the alternative? You don't like your body, and you can't fathom saying, "I love you" to a bulging belly and flabby thighs. You've heard of the stand-in-front-of-the-mirror-naked exercise and *you ain't goin' there!* Besides, you think telling your body you love it as is would be condoning the condition you're in or saying it's okay to stay fat, or wrinkled, or scarred, or whatever scarlet letter you have painted on your chest right now. Accepting your body won't help you get into better shape, lose weight, or eat healthy, right?

Wrong. The birthplace of good self-care, especially physical fitness, is a positive and loving relationship with your body. When you're operating out of love, or plain respect, for your body, you can't help but take good care of it. If you purchase a new car or dress you absolutely love, you treat it with gentleness and care. You wouldn't take your new Austin Martin off-roading, and you wouldn't put a silk "dry clean only" dress through the washer and dryer. You protect and nurture the things you value.

Perhaps you have children in your care. The responsibility of nurturing a child requires that you operate out of love and respect for that little person. You wouldn't feed a child candy for dinner every day or forcibly keep him awake all night. The same is true with your body: when you love and value your body, you treat it with respect. Stop buying into the beauty box idea that you need to hate yourself into shape or you can change your behavior via self-loathing. Loathing your figure won't build a decent self-care practice, won't help you change your behavior, and won't make you love yourself, ever.

If loving your body right now feels like too far of a stretch, aim to respect your body. Keep in mind the unlimited number of things your body does all day every day to keep you alive. Your heart pumps tirelessly twenty-four hours a day, your entire life. Hormones, oxygen, and proteins never stop circulating to keep your body in perfect homeostasis. Your immune system patrols around the clock to ward off threatening entities. Mankind, with our ever-increasing resources and knowledge, can't begin to build anything in the likeness of you—we can barely create a replacement part or change the body's "oil"! Your body is a bundle of phenomenal interactions every minute of every day. At least respect it as the miraculous organism it is.

When healthy eating comes out of respect for your body's health and longevity, it will come easier. As exercise grows into a moving meditation for your body and medication for your mind, it will become a desire. Moving into a mind-state of love and respect for your body—a loving marriage—is the best guarantee for a healthy and fit body you'll ever have.

After all, loving your body is your natural state of being. Young children love their bodies no matter how they look, because they don't know they shouldn't. Only when a child has been exposed to images, ideas, comments, and beliefs about what a body *should* look like—what society finds attractive and valuable—does she began to judge and criticize herself. When she gets her prescription filled by the same optometrist you did, the hate begins.

Think of the last time you held, bathed, or changed a baby. Did it occur to you that the child's body was "imperfect" by society's standards? Did you think her cheeks were too puffy or her butt too small? Were you disgusted that her belly was round or her thighs rippled with cellulite? Was her semi-grown-in hair abhorrent? I doubt it.

Infants are absolutely beautiful, perfect little humans. Their waist circumference far out measures their hips, their cheeks resemble a chipmunk in the fall, their heads can be a scaly, balding mess, and they're flanked with cellulite! Nonetheless, they are magnificent. They are gorgeous! An infant or young child doesn't know she's out of proportion, or that her fat stores or skin aren't ideal. She simply is; she lives in her body as if it were the carriage of her soul and a means for her to experience the world. Her energy about her body is neutral until we teach her otherwise.

So, what happened between your last diaper change and your thirty-eighth birthday that made your body so disgusting? Why is your matured body any less physically precious than when you were an infant? Why do you think it's okay to say things about your body that you wouldn't be caught dead saying about a child? I would guess that you have less caterpillar rolls on your thighs today than at nine months old. Isn't your head less scaly and your body more proportioned? You have teeth now, right? It's your perspective that's askew from drinking beauty box Kool-Aid©!

The truth is that your body is neutral; it's your thoughts about it that are ugly, fat, and old. You're that same pure magnificence that you were as an infant. Your body is still that perfect and beautiful little creature, only bigger. Your body is precious—*as it is*—just like an infant's. Babies are proof that a belly, jowls, toothless-ness, and cellulite are neutral or beautiful and absolutely lovable when you're wearing love-colored glasses. One of the reasons children are so beautiful is that they know they're perfect as they are and consequently exude that energy. Their energy has nothing to do with looks; their energy is present in authentic being-ness, a.k.a. love.

Changing the lenses with which you see yourself is a choice to think differently. Decide how you would like to think and feel about your body. Which of your beliefs are old, fat, ugly, or simply not serving you? What would you like to believe, think, and feel about your body? Aim to think of your body as if it were a child's: perfect and lovable. When you touch, talk, or think about your body, do so as if it were that innocent vessel of life and purity as a child would think of herself.

As you begin to think differently about your body, you'll shift your energy or vibration about your body. One of the best ways to stimulate an energy and thought shift is through gratitude. Get grateful for your body as is, right now. Begin to think about which parts of your physical self you're grateful for possessing or experiencing. What parts or systems of your body are functioning perfectly today? There are millions of processes happening this very moment, of which you're likely unaware, keeping you alive and healthy. You've probably been blessed with a healthy, functioning body for so long that you've become spoiled about it. When was the last time you took a spin around a hospital? Walked through a floor or two lately and considered bitching about your thighs? You could try sitting on the bed of someone in intensive care and pinch the fat rolls on your belly to get her rating on the foulness of your physique. I think you'd be asked to leave. Gratitude is the bridge to love and reality.

You can help what you think, in fact you choose what to think and believe. If Victor Frankl can decide he's not a prisoner in a Nazi concentration camp, and Claire Wineland can maintain a positive perspective as a teen with cystic fibrosis, you can make a tiny thought choice to like your thighs or stop berating your belly. The next chapter offers more ideas on how to change your body beliefs.

⌘ **Mental Fitness Exercise:** Infantilize your body. Think of your physical body as if it were a small child. Write your child body a love note from the mommy you, and tell her all the wonderful things about her body: how her body is healthy and strong, beautiful and precious, etc., as it is.

⌘ **Mental Fitness Exercise:** How would you buck the societal point of view if you could? How would you change the beauty box optometric Rx? Would you like to see women who look like you or someone you know walk runways, fill magazines, and become sex symbols?

⌘ **Mental Fitness Exercise:** Start a body gratitude journal. Every night or morning enter at least five things about your physical self you're grateful for, especially focusing on non-appearance items. For instance, you can write: my heart beating regularly or 172,000 times today, my immune system taking care of inflammation and bacteria in my gut, etc. Get the picture? If you get stuck get Og Mandino's *The Greatest Miracle in the World* for some ideas.

🖱 Go to www.loveyourselffit.com/inspiration for a downloadable version of these exercises.

CHAPTER 14

Shifting Your Perception: The Tools

"I refuse to think of them as chin hairs.
I think of them as stray eyebrows."

Janette Barber

Throughout this book you're asked to shift your perception or look at a subject from a different angle. Even your bathroom mirror has a new identity and name! This chapter delves into the thought systems we use to form our beliefs and offers several tools to redirect your perspective.

A belief system is the set of thoughts you accept as true about any given aspect of existence. They're your interpretations of reality, the way you see the world. Beliefs are formed from your perceptions, experiences, upbringing, environment, relationships, society, and your self-talk (internal dialogue), and they're ingrained by continued thought investment. Together, your collective belief systems make up your state of mind.

As well, your belief systems influence your perception, i.e., *what* you see.

For example, if in your life experience you've only seen red apples, you'll probably come to believe that all apples are red. Perhaps your society idolizes extremely lean bodies; then you would come to believe only very lean bodies are ideal. If you hold a strong belief, particularly one with an emotional charge behind it, you'll be convinced of its reality. Unconsciously, you'll not only seek evidence to support your belief systems, you'll find it.

The energy of emotion has a glue-like quality to it when it comes to your cognitive reality. Emotionally charged beliefs and feelings, especially those established under duress, tend to sear into one's consciousness. This is why you remember events that were dramatic, frightening, or painful. A car accident, dog bite, or being teased as a child are hard to forget, because your brain is wired to make you remember things that are scary or painful. You may have an aversion to tequila or an unreasonable fear of small spaces for similar reasons. Avoiding threatening or damaging people, animals, and situations was helpful for your ancestral cavewomen's survival. It's survival HTML code for your brain.

Additionally, the more frequently you entertain a line of thought, the more ingrained it becomes physiologically. Imagine your brain is like a field of grass. The more often you walk a path the more prominent that path becomes. Your brain continues to recruit neurons to thicken the areas of the brain that are most often used. Or you can think of repetitious thought as weight lifting for your brain. The more often you think something, the more powerful it becomes. Adored or feared, when you hold a belief near and dear to your consciousness, it will become the buffest, most well-fed neural avenue in your brain.

As we've learned from PNI, your mind lives in each cell of your body, not just in brain cells. The beliefs you hold are carried out and held in every single cell of your entire body. Knowing this, what do you think your negative or non-supportive beliefs are doing to your fitness or weight loss attempts? Your posture? Your immune system? Your digestion? Being stuck with an abusive and unloving person is a miserable way to live and it's affecting your physiology. So knock it off!

Think of your mind as a computer. It's reprogrammable; it's fluid and flexible. In fact, you can change your mind in an instant. A compelling story, new facts and figures, or a vivid thirty-second experience can immediately change your opinion about a subject or event. A terrifying news report of burglaries in your neighborhood from door-to-door salesmen, followed by a knock on the door can send your heart racing. Just as well, long-term, low level input can alter your perceptions and beliefs about a subject. The reason you're so judgmental of your appearance is repetitive conditioning. I'm sure you could list foods that contribute to belly fat just from the magazines you've fingered through over the last couple of years. Be it long-term consistency or emotionally charged facts, changing your mind is the most powerful way to shift your energy and behavior, and subsequently your life.

We've already determined we need a shift in perspective and that this perspective is programmable. It's your job to program your neurons with daily doses of clear, kind conditioning. Every morning, each day, choose what you would like to think about your body and relationship, your beauty or grace, and remind yourself of them throughout the day. Repetition is your belief and energy gear shifter. Consistent, directed input will change your mind and your body will follow.

You need to challenge a muscle regularly to make it stronger, or change its functionality or appearance. You know this. Reading the brilliant writing of this chapter one time isn't likely going to shift you—even though it's the most amazing and mind-blowing thing you've ever read! (I'm being silly of course.) You need to shift yourself by starting to think of your mind and thoughts as muscles that improve your perspective. This is your next and most important step in building your loving relationship: a daily exercise of challenging old thoughts or the healthy input of affirmative brain food. This is a game changer. Your level of consistency with your new perspective input will determine your feelings, thoughts, and energy—then physiology—of your body and self-care. Remember: redirect, praise, repeat.

Use the following Mental Fitness Exercises to help shift your mindset and energy. Your thought choices are muscle builders for body-mind relationship: where your mind leads, your body follows!

⌘ **Mental Fitness Exercise:** Assess your beliefs. On a piece of paper write out at least three body, food, or exercise related beliefs. Take a look at your beliefs. Be honest with yourself. Are your beliefs supporting you, or are they setting you up for failure and self-loathing? Ask yourself: is this thought grown of fear or love? Be aware of your energy when you're mentally chewing on a subject. If your vibration feels off or negative, you're probably coming from your little-i self and your thoughts beg to be questioned.

⌘ **Mental Fitness Exercise:** Choose new beliefs to install. Thoughts change feelings. Make affirmative statements that are true and that make you feel good. Then make these new beliefs official: write them down; claim them; input them throughout the day or as needed with self-talk, affirmations, pictures, affirmative reading, and audio of the same vein. "Redirect, praise, repeat" will do you no good unless you have the "redirect" part ready to go when you need it. If your current belief system includes stuff about how fat or old your body is, how hard it is for you to resist sweets, or that you used to be so much more attractive when you_____, then decide those are B.S.! Those types of beliefs aren't helpful or sup-portive, and most importantly, they don't create good feelings around your body, food, or self-care. They are commentary from the abusive, loser boyfriend. "I am radiant, healthy, and gorgeous at my age" or "It is so easy for me to listen to my body now." Try "I eat with the Zen-like ju-ju of a Buddhist monk" or "God, I just keep getting better looking every day—in fact, I can't wait to see how hot I look tomorrow!" Aren't those better feeling thoughts? And who's to say they're less true than the crap you've been preaching to yourself? What if there is something to this and all that negative self-talk is making this body thing harder? Create an internal environment (and clear reminder in your external environment) that supports your new loving marriage with your body.

⌘ **Mental Fitness Exercise:** Take an input inventory. Monitor the external input your mind receives each day. Like a computer, your mind receives input and produces corresponding output. What are you feeding your mind? Is what you're watching on TV, reading, listening to, and talking about nurturing the beauty box or your authentic self? Decrease your exposure to negative, body-hating input and replace it with meaningful, worthwhile input. Subscribe to different magazines, surround yourself with like-minded people, or change the channel. You are solely responsible for what you intellectually eat.

⌘ **Mental Fitness Exercise:** Alter your self-talk. Self-talk is your inner dialogue; it's what you say to yourself when no one else is talking. Self-talk consists of anything you say to yourself: interpretations, observations, opinions, judgments, and reactions. Your self-talk challenges or validates your beliefs. Beliefs are greatly amplified by the words you say to yourself repeatedly—recall your weight lifting neurons. Self-talk is an enormous factor in how you feel about your body. Do you encourage yourself like a loving parent would do, or do you adopt the belittling attitude of an abusive spouse? Pretend you're the most positive, loving, awesome mom in the world and parent your body. If you don't know how, just make it up. Adjust your self-talk to the kind that expresses unconditional, positive regard and a supportive, nurturing partnership. Repeat this kind of self-talk until it becomes habit. In fact, go on a negative self-talk diet. Three weeks of no bitch-in-the-mirror judgmental flap! I challenge you to a positive self-talk duel!

⌘ **Mental Fitness Exercise:** Use affirmations and visualization. An affirmation is a statement affirming a condition as if it already exists. It's best if it uses the present tense and is stated positively. This is guided self-talk with the intention to stimulate a feeling. For example, instead of saying "I'm not fat," say "I'm fit and healthy" or "I'm getting fitter every day". Keep it simple and easy to remember. Create a few optimal affirmations to work with at a time. The world has been writing your affirmations for decades, so it's time to write some for yourself. Simply think about the affirmative energy you want to create and write it as is. But the feeling or image it creates in your mind is the most important part about it. It must seed the feeling or energy you want to live in.

Visualization is a psychological tool utilized for many purposes, from getting over a cold to getting over a high jump. It's used extensively in sports psychology. You can use visualization for any situation, dilemma, or goal, whether you're dealing with a presentation at work, remodeling your bathroom, or bench pressing two hundred pounds. The only way to use affirmations and visualizations is with energetic conviction—meaning emotional charge or energy. Put yourself into a scene or an experience with emotional energy. Your "I feel great exercising" affirmation would be accompanied by closing your eyes and picturing yourself effortlessly running down the beach, feeling fit and energized, breathing easily, and feeling your leg muscles working. Imagine yourself drinking water after your run, feeling so good and refreshed. Focus on how you feel and what you're thinking. Replay it often. Imag-spiration!

⌘ **Mental Fitness Exercise:** Cue yourself! Continue to remind yourself of your intentions with visual cues. Cues are useful implements to keep you focused while initiating change in thoughts or behaviors. They can be visual reminders that support your goals—from sticky notes, to pictures, photos, collages, recordings, or videos. It's a good idea to put reminders in places you frequent, like the bathroom mirror, the wall in front of the toilet, the refrigerator door, your electronic screens, or even the steering wheel of your car. Make sure they stimulate the energy, essence, or content you want to experience. Another type of cue worth mentioning is the negative type; those things that conjure up or remind you of the war with weight, or that stimulate a little-i need to measure some body part or the sum of its parts. Bail your scale. If you need help, watch the movie *Office Space* and take some pointers on how to ceremoniously destroy a mechanical device to rap music. The only person who should be weighing you, talking about numbers, or measuring any part of your physical self is your doctor or physical therapist. (A personal trainer checking for limb discrepancies gets a pass for that only.) But really, what do you think when you see a scale? "Oh goodie! Yay, yay, yay!" Or "Oh crap. Maybe if I take off my bra too…oh crap!" When you weigh yourself it doesn't matter, measure, or reflect anything about what you're doing towards health, strength, longevity, fitness, nutrition, alignment, believing in yourself, or living your values. You want to measure, because you think a number will give you the essence, feeling, or experience of being fit, but it doesn't. It indiscriminately ewards or punishes you. It takes one, infinitesimally small aspect of one tiny part of your soul's carriage and measures it for purposes of judgment, comparison, or ego. How does that help you get it or put it together to live and love with your body, food, or self-care? It doesn't. Scales, calipers, and the like are weapons of the war. Keep them only if you want to keep fighting.

⌘ **Mental Fitness Exercise:** Watch your mouth. The words you use with regularity help shape your beliefs, energy, and body-mind. They are a reflection of your inner dialog and direct your focus. Replace the words hate or war with peace ("I'm at peace with my thighs" vs. "I hate my thighs"), the word weight with lean ("I'm leaning out" instead of "I'm trying to lose weight"), and so on. The words you choose can have a powerful impact on your psyche and the minds of those around you, like your children.

Affirmations, pictures, visualizations, and any other tools you use should feel good authentically. Your goal in using these is to conjure up the feeling—the vibration or energy—of the belief or goal. Avoid pictures, photos, or words that challenge you from a little-i perspective. Use nothing that invokes the energy of longing, jealousy, resentment, or guilt. You want to put yourself into an attractive state of being, actualizing instead of resisting your goals. The feeling of wanting, envy, remorse, needing, and resentment are repulsive energies. Instead use attractive energies with a positive or loving vibration or feeling. Some examples would be confidence during a presentation, relaxation walking into your newly remodeled bathroom, or ease in executing that two hundred pound bench press. The essence of what you want to experience—confidence, relaxation, or ease—is what you truly want, so that's your focus in your shifting or programming efforts.

The last place fitness shows itself is in your physical body. Whatever type of training, conditioning, sport, hobby, or event anyone partakes in, and however she goes about executing that movement, self-presentation, or fitness level, *it always happens in the mind first.* Conscious choice is one of your greatest gifts. Use it.

Go to www.loveyourselffit.com/inspiration for a downloadable version of these exercises.

SECTION V

Healthy Ever After:
The Practice

CHAPTER 15

A Wedding or a Marriage? Choosing a LTR

"Marriage is not a noun; it's a verb. It isn't something you get.
It's something you do. It's the way you love your partner every day."

Barbara De Angelis

Do you remember dreaming about your wedding day? (Queue music…) Planning the ceremony, picturing your husband-to-be waiting at the altar, and picking "your colors" all sound familiar to a starry-eyed young romantic. Most girls grow up fantasizing about the day they'll say "I do" and ride off into the sunset with Mr. Wonderful.

All the dreaming and planning never prepares you for the reality of a marriage, because your wedding day does not a marriage make! A wedding is simply the official and/or public declaration of the start of a contract between two people. Likewise, achieving your goal weight or size is not the reality of being fit; it's an official number or destination point, like your wedding day. Twelve percent body fat is not a state of being, it's a measurement. You believe that once you get there, it's all good. But states of being must be cultivated from an ongoing practice. Whether it's being fit or being happily married, neither becomes reality until you make the ongoing commitment to the daily practice of it. Therefore, your first step to creating healthy ever after is turning your fitness outcome fantasy into a real daily practice.

Arrival thinking is deeply ingrained in our society. We believe that when one reaches a certain marker or goal, it means she's arrived at and will remain in a state of success. Reaching the goal becomes the primary focus under the guise that achieving the goal will bring a lasting internal experience. "I'm sorry Dave, I'm afraid I can't do that." (HAL 9000 from *2001: A Space Odyssey*) Reaching a location, like a space station with an attitude, doesn't equate with staying in that location. In other words, arriving doesn't mean squat. It's lovely when you reach your goal weight, but in reality it has as much longevity as a day-old marriage. Talk to me when you've maintained it for three or four years. Your wedding day might be gorgeous, and reaching your goal weight is awesome, but neither is happily ever after. Rejoice in it, celebrate, and then return to your practice. Otherwise, when you hold onto arrival thinking and you reach your goal, you'll stop the practice part that got you there! Haven't you seen this happen with actual couples or your own weight loss saga?

Using arrival thinking for a long-term commitment always leads to struggle, extremes, and a vicious cycle of guilt and failure. You remember all too well how the cycle goes: it starts with that spandex and sequins thing. You envision yourself with the perfect body, draped strategically among the skinny bitches at your Bunco group, or perhaps trotting down some tropical beach while frisbee-playing men stumble over themselves attempting to get a look at you. Blah, blah, blah and your dream window slams shut with a glimpse of your reflection and a snide remark from you-know-who. Your argument with the mirror bitch is followed with an emotionally charged self-improvement declaration, complete with a drastic broccolini and brown rice diet amendment and forty-two hours of exercise a week. You know you just flipped the crazy switch, because to you it sounds realistic and well thought out. Before you know it you're on Diet Row again, set up to fail and recycle through the same painful ordeal *again*. Each time you add weight to yourself, both on the scale and in the psyche.

Also recall that you never quite get "there". Body builders are a perfect example of this principle. Ego always wants more; there's always someone richer, more beautiful, more successful, or more muscular. As soon as you achieve everything you've strived for, you'll want more. Think about it. When you were at your very thinnest or the high point of your youthful beauty, did you think you were thin or pretty enough? Have you ever received a large sum of money and thought, "That's enough, I don't want any more"? Or have you ever gotten *everything* done on your entire to-do list? I don't think so! Considering that your little-i will always be little, it will never have enough. It constantly needs more to feel equal and therefore becomes insatiable.

Remember: arrival thinking works great when you're cleaning out your closet or painting your house. Even when faced with a longer-term project like college or a difficult pregnancy, it can be useful. Only when the task at hand can be completed within a measurable term, has to be done once, or can be participated in occasionally, does destination based thinking work well.

For the long-term things you do daily, arrival thinking is fallible. Taking good care of yourself lies in the long-term category. Choosing not to have fast food, munch on office goodies, or eat huge portions requires conscious awareness and aligned choices habitually. Getting enough rest, exercising regularly, and meeting your spiritual needs are all ongoing processes that require a consistent practice and mind-state.

Practice Thinking

When you ignore the process it becomes uncomfortable and sometimes miserable. Hooking up with an abusive jerk is an awful experience and doesn't make for long-term bliss. Depriving yourself of enjoyable foods or forcing hours of unpleasant exercise every week is an experience you can do without and doesn't make for long-term bliss.

Yet when it comes to fitness we rarely consider the road to our destination, because we're so fixated on the end result. We have a low tolerance for discomfort and a seeming inability to delay gratification. We get angry in traffic, impatient with our waitresses, and we want pills that will cure our ills overnight. We want results immediately—as if we can jump from desire to fulfillment without thought or an experience of the path between.

Fitness is not immediate. The last place it manifests is in your physique! It's an ongoing process and it never ends, therefore it must be palatable. You can't sign up for a forty-five-minute daily commute that makes you angry every day and expect to arrive happy and contented. You either change jobs, find another route, or entertain yourself with better thoughts while you're sitting in traffic. Your self-care is similar: you either change what you're doing, find another way to do what you need to do, or entertain yourself while you're doing it. You're the one who can turn it into something you can do every day; otherwise don't expect it to last or be happy about it.

Can you imagine if you applied the same erroneous logic you've been using with self-care to other commitments in your life? Say you finally get the job you've been longing for after months of courting an employer. Does this mean you've achieved professional success, your career is complete, and you'll never have to put in another day at the office? Perhaps you've conceived a child. Does this mean your role as a parent is over and you have no further responsibilities? Sound unrealistic? So is the notion that once you starve yourself into your ideal dress size you've magically made it a lifelong habit.

Fitness is a series of decisions you make every day. Being fit is like being a parent or employee. When your child is born, your role as a parent is just beginning. An entire lifetime of everyday decisions and responsibilities lie ahead. It's the same with a new career. Once you land a job in the field of your choice, you've only started on the road to becoming successful, not arrived there. The day you get your dream job is the same day your work begins. It may take ten to twenty years of daily commitment before you're considered "successful" and establish yourself fully in the business world.

Anything in life that has meaning or substance requires regular maintenance. Your house demands the upkeep of structure, landscaping, utilities, maintenance, and cleanliness, not to mention a mortgage and taxes. Your plants and yard need water, sunlight, good soil, pest control, and nutrients. If you have a hobby or collection, you may spend countless hours and possibly large amounts of money to maintain your passion. Even your pubic hair requires maintenance; trim it or play *Jumanji*—the jungle game—you choose. Every long-term relationship, be it with your children, spouse, or friends, necessitates contact, nurturing, and communication, or else it will dissipate.

What makes you think that fitness is any different? Are your eating habits and inclinations fixable by a prescribed breakfast-lunch-dinner chart? Will your disdain for exercise be solved by a flashy workout gadget? Will your body judging cease with enough cosmetic procedures?

Fitness can't be handled like a temp job or a babysitting gig. If you think "being fit" is an arrival point, you'll never fully arrive. Meeting your fitness goals is just the beginning, merely one of the steps along your path. There is no arriving. You're in process with your self-care right now. You've never been out of this process.

Nice theory, but how do you switch from arrival thinking to practice thinking? Practice thinking is a series of small, simple decisions you make every day, just as you would maintaining your marriage, job, or home. Use the tools you've learned to reprogram your mental computer and support yourself: The Work, CORE technique, and all the perception shifting tools in Chapter 14. Clear out the blocks to loving your body. Redirect your puppy-mind when it's crapping all over your living room floor, and allow your sacred time and space to emerge. (The next two chapters will also assist you in practice thinking.)

After all, life is not about arrival at a set destination and neither is consistent self-care. Your life doesn't wait to happen until you reach a certain magical age. Nor will it climax the day you die. Your self-care, too, will not reach its pinnacle the day you achieve your ideal weight, nor end the day you "fall off the wagon". Life is about every day and so is self-care. Neither is about getting there; both are about being here today.

⌘ **Mental Fitness Exercise:** Which areas of your life have you managed brilliantly? Which aspects of your relationships, career, parenting, etc., do you feel good about or manage daily without much trouble? What is your train of thought in this area? How do you think about it? Are you more patient with your kids because their brains are developing, or do you have no problem consistently kicking ass in your career? Take note of the areas where you're naturally using practice thinking, and investigate your thought habits so you can use the same thought habits with self-care.

⌘ **Mental Fitness Exercise:** Use the answers from the above exercise to creatively construct a new process-oriented mindset in regards to self-care. For example, if you're gentle on kids because you understand they're still developing, then how can you be gentler on yourself when it comes to exercise or self-talk? If you're extremely persistence with your work, how can you use that same drive to move you with self-care? Which ways are you calming, succeeding, or inspiring yourself that you can duplicate with your exercise, eating, and being kind to yourself?

Go to www.loveyourselffit.com/inspiration for a downloadable version of these exercises.

CHAPTER 16

The Flow Zone: Your Fitness Nirvana

"To heal is to make happy."

A Course in Miracles

I magine your girlfriend Teresa has signed up for the new gym that opened in town. It's super cool, with all new equipment and a staff of young, hard-bodied professionals. Teresa had a baby three months ago and has been unable to lose more than a few pounds. She feels a bit intimidated her first day at the gym, surrounded by strange equipment, body builders, and loud music. But she forces herself to go because she's made a commitment to lose this weight by New Year's Eve.

Swallowing her pride, Teresa dons her spandex and shows up for her first complimentary training appointment with Bruce. Bruce puts Teresa through a workout and encourages her to cut calories and carbs from her diet. Teresa leaves, agreeing to return to the gym tomorrow. When morning arrives, she's sore, tired, and thoroughly uninspired to go to the gym; however, she forces herself to return again. Unfortunately for Teresa, her second day is much the same as the first: she feels uncomfortable, intimidated, and uninspired to return.

How long would you give Teresa's new exercise commitment? What are her chances for success? If you guessed between slim and none, you're right. Most people don't maintain an exercise program beyond a couple of months.[10] The majority have no idea how to set up or maintain a long-term practice, particularly if it's unpleasant.

Teresa is a perfect example of arrival thinking, or thinking of her fitness as a destination to be reached instead of a life-long relationship. She's been swept up by her destination-based goal, and she believes that extrinsic motivation will get and keep her on track. She signed up for a type of exercise that doesn't inspire or attract her, and she feels intimidated by the whole gym scene. She's forcing herself to show up from guilt, obligation, and a "have-to" mentality.

If you were looking for a mate in his late forties who enjoys hiking and Bach, would you go to a nightclub full of twenty-somethings or to spring break in Cabo San Lucas? Maybe if you want to play cougar! But otherwise, no. You wouldn't go to places you don't want to be: you would look for a mate your speed, someplace you'd want to be, like a classical concert or trail hiking club. Similarly with fitness, seek a love for fitness where you're likely to find it: where your interests lie. Your ideal fitness or self-care will flow, meaning it will be easy and feel good or natural as you undertake it each day. Flow can be defined as a movement, continuation, or stream, an outpouring or abundance, and these are exactly the words to associate with your self-care: continuing, abundant, movement. This is the next step in creating happily-ever-healthy: finding flow with your daily fitness practice.

Anyone beginning a fitness endeavor must create flow for herself. If previous fitness programs or diets had flowed for you, you wouldn't be challenged with finding a new solution now. Most diets and exercise programs will work when you stay with them. However, you usually stop practicing the prescribed behaviors and then resume your former level of fitness because it lacked flow, among other things. Flow is part of the glue that keeps the everyday practice palatable and long lasting. Self-care that has no glue won't stick for you!

So, how do you find flow with the physical part of fitness and make it an enjoyable process every day? How do you make it effortless when it seems like torture? What's going to make it feasible for you over the long term?

One of the most effective principles for staying in process with self-care is what I call the "flow zone". The flow zone comprises of your personal parameters for keeping fitness a practice. These parameters are a way to make your self-care goals a reality right now. The flow zone is the balanced middle between the polar ends of the extremes: bingeing sloth and fitness fanatic.

Those of us challenged by fitness have a pattern of swinging from one end of the behavior zone to the other, exercising or being slothful without ever finding a balance. The flow zone is the middle, where you can hold your self-care in a functional place. The flow zone means you're living a healthy *and* enjoyable lifestyle day after day without resistance or feeling deprived. Contrary to yo-yoing on a diet or going on and off an exercise program, you create a natural, smooth flow in the middle.

Think of yourself as a pendulum. On each end of your arc are two behavioral extremes: couch potato or fitness freak. When you pull yourself to one end of the behavioral extreme, like a pendulum you'll swing back to the other extreme. A hard-core diet will always lead to a hard-core binge. Overexerting in the gym will force you to compensate with extra rest or by nursing injuries. When the latest extreme fix doesn't work, your pendulum swings back to its opposite end and leads you to more extreme programs, more failures, and finally negative psycho-emotional consequences.

When you pull your self-care to one extreme, it will always swing back with additional momentum to the other extreme. Too much in either direction will cause an imbalance.

The flow zone is heavenly. It's the answer to extremes—a place in the very center of your self-care pendulum's arc. Ideally, you'll find a zone in which you can remain balanced, one that allows you to have the food and movement you enjoy without compromising your health or your goals. The flow zone is about living with balance and staying aligned in a way that's sustainable.

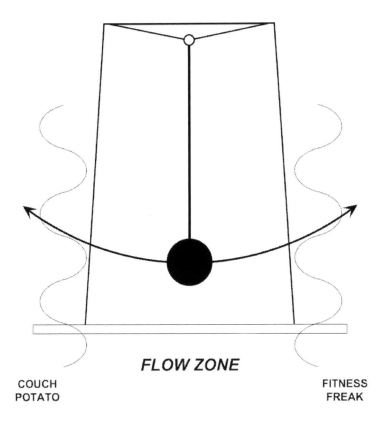

FLOW ZONE

COUCH
POTATO

FITNESS
FREAK

Living in the flow zone is actually quite simple. For example, when planning a meal consider not only your healthiest choices, but also what would taste best to you. Good self-care includes foods you enjoy. Ask yourself, "How can I make this meal healthier and more enjoyable?" How about adding a salad or vegetables? Can you forgo the butter or cream dressing for an avocado- or yogurt-based sauce? Can you have whole-grain bread instead of white? Can you exchange the dessert for fruit or have a cup of delicious hot tea instead? Ask yourself, "What will make me healthier and stay aligned with my meaningful goals?" Health is queen! Using this flow zone technique, you'll fare brilliantly—much better than an all-or-nothing plan of extremes.

Thinking with the flow zone mindset will move you closer to your goals and allow you to maintain a healthy lifestyle you can live with. I imagine you're thinking, "But what about real life? How the heck do I stay in the flow zone when I have work, kids, and softball pizza parties to go to?" Easy, just be creative! Imagine that after a long day at work you must take your son's little league team out for pizza. You're hungry and you love pizza, but you're trying to eat healthy and lean out (a.k.a. lose fat). How can you stay in the flow zone and enjoy a healthy meal? *Can you have your pizza and eat it too?*

Yes! You can have one slice of pizza and a salad, instead of three pieces of pizza and a soda. Or you can wrap up three pieces of pizza and save them for your scheduled "free" eating day. You can choose a low-fat, veggie-laden sandwich or pasta with red sauce. You can ask your hubby to meet you at the pizza place to take over so you can go home and eat an organic, whole grain pizza. There are lots of ways to handle this situation in a way that will satisfy your appetite while maintaining a healthy, balanced, yet yummy zone.

You can make any situation healthier. You can sit up straighter in your chair right now and contract your abdominals to support your back. At the grocery store don't just park far away but bring your cart back. Walk the response to your coworker that you were going to e-mail. If you don't have time to go to the gym, walk your dog before dinner or cruise around your office building for ten minutes at ten and three o'clock. Exercise in small increments can be just as effective as longer sessions. Ten minutes three times a day is as good as thirty minutes straight. (Some researchers are experimenting with even smaller doses of exercise, for example three, twenty-second bursts of high intensity cardio, with interesting results.) Simply ask yourself, "How can I move my body more today?"

The flow zone is based on the principle that *everything counts*. Everything you do, think, avoid, or say to yourself each day counts to make you healthier and fitter, or the opposite. Author Adelle Davis said, "Every day you choose to either build health or disease in yourself." She's right. Your choices today will move you in a healthier direction or an unhealthier direction. The same is true about tomorrow and the next day. The flow zone is the positive place where you can be satisfied *and* your body can be healthier. When you find yourself faced with a self-care decision, slow down, take a couple of deep breaths, and remind yourself that every little thing you do toward better health counts.

If you make a choice you wish you hadn't, don't clobber yourself afterward with guilt and "I blew it!" thinking. Attempting to compensate with extreme thinking and pendulous behavior pulls you off center and into separation, abusiveness, and arriving. Author and eating guru Geneen Roth says, "For every diet there is an equal and opposite binge." Remind yourself of what pendulous choices do to your self-care. Return to the happy medium of the flow zone, and be mindful that this is a process. There's no place to get to; everything you do always counts, positive or negative. So, if you catch yourself five cookies into a ten-cookie bender, stop. Put them away and know that you just took a huge step in a loving direction! One less cookie is a winning step toward the flow zone, and five less is a giant leap.

Any relationship has lows and highs, dips and peaks. Fitness, just like your relationships, has ups and downs. Sometimes you'll be better at staying in your flow zone than other times. Just like parenting or your career, it's the bigger picture of consistently good self-care over time that will keep you fit and healthy. Little slips and dips won't break you as long as you continue to return to the healthy center zone.

For example, holidays or travel often present eating and time challenges that leave you with several self-care dips in a row. This is reality, and you have to allow your self-care flow through all the seasons of life. Therefore, figure out a way to take the best possible care of your body you can manage during dips or challenging times. Your self-care isn't going to be perfect all the time, so don't to waste your energy on self-flagellation. Bring your puppy-mind back to the newspaper, and put your mind and energy into going-with-the-flow zone.

The flow zone is also a call to "Lighten up Francis!" as Sergeant Hooka said in the movie *Stripes*. Lighten up your thinking, or attachment to the idea that fitness or leaning out has to be a chore or major endeavor. Just watch children play for a few minutes, and it will be evident that movement is fun, normal, and natural for our species. Moving your body, paying attention to its cues, and allowing it to be what it innately is (without a bunch of your shouldy, psycho-emotional crap piled on it), is one of the most freeing things you can do! You can have a blast building strength, balance, and flexibility when you change your mind about it.

Adding fun to your self-care equation is simple. Think light. Think fun. What would make movement fun for you? Music or people? Dance class or outdoor yoga? Maybe random water sports in the summer and likewise with the frozen stuff in the winter. Can you watch comedians on your DVR while you're stretching? Be silly and have fun seeking out playful ways to move your body. Lightening up is a big move toward lightening up!

Start flowing in the zone right this minute. And if you slip up, start flowing again. There is no starting tomorrow. Your body has always been and will continue to be in the flow zone called homeostasis. It's what your body naturally does. Centered and flowing is the most natural state of being for your spirit's RV.

⌘ **Mental Fitness Exercise:** What does your flow zone look like? Define moderate parameters for yourself—where's your edge on either side? How will flow manifest in your self-care? Be specific about your daily experience of easy, enjoyable, and fun movement, eating, and lifestyle. If everything counts, what can you say to yourself to keep your thinking in the flow zone?

⌘ **Mental Fitness Exercise:** How can you lighten up and make this more fun? List five fun ways to move your body.

Go to www.loveyourselffit.com/inspiration for a downloadable version of these exercises.

CHAPTER 17

HEED:
Your Flow Zone Guide

*"It (the body) will be strong and healthy if the mind does not abuse it
by assigning to it roles it cannot fill, to purposes beyond its scope, and to
exalted aims which it cannot accomplish."*

A Course in Miracles

very situation offers you an opportunity to make better
self-care choices through thought or deed. There are four simple
guidelines you can use to help you keep your mind centered in
the flow zone: HEED.

HEED is an acronym for *healthy, enjoyable, effective, and doable.* The
HEED acronym works to remind you to pause prior to any self-care
choice and literally heed the flow zone principles. Using the HEED
principles will help you stay in the flow zone with your self-care, and you
might be able to guess that I'm going to say it's "the next step" in your
happily-ever-healthy.

Healthy

If your practice is to be considered self-care it must be *healthy*. If your daily routine isn't healthy for body, mind, and spirit, then it's not really self-care.

Healthy is a subjective term. You probably have you own idea of what being healthy means. The medical and fitness industries each have their own definitions of, and measuring sticks for, "health". I have my own ideas as well. For instance, I believe health is not the absence of disease or a low body-fat percentage, rather an optimum state of being for the body, mind, and spirit. Health enables the highest level of function for all parts of the self. Being healthy often demands action and sometimes discomfort, but it doesn't harm or injure. Being healthy feels great, renders freedom, and emanates love for your whole self.

Using health as one of your flow zone guidelines will keep your focus on "good health" instead of "weight loss". When you focus on fat or weight, that's what expands in your consciousness. *Thoughts are energy, and what you put your energy into grows.* Think of your mental energy as a laser beam. Wherever you focus this laser beam will fill with energy. Keep your energy focused on what you want more of, like health, good posture, or self-love.

If you aim for good health, your weight will balance itself. Research shows that people who make their goal "good health" maintain weight loss more effectively than those who aspire purely to weight loss.[11,12] Striving for health will never sabotage you or hinder your wellbeing.

You can use this flow zone principle for any area of your life. Ask yourself what a healthy body means to you. What makes a relationship healthy? How can you make your finances healthier? Health is a principle that can be used to enhance any area of your life, and it's the source of fitness.

Enjoyable

The second HEED principle is *enjoyment*. Your everyday lifestyle must be a design that is enjoyable to you. Hello: if you don't like it, you're not going to eat it, drink it, or do it! If your daily requirements aren't appetizing to you, you'll be unable to maintain them long term.

A perfect example is the high protein diet craze. High protein diets are not my idea of healthy, but they do enable weight loss. Nonetheless, most people find them hard to stick with for long. Our bodies and brains crave carbohydrates; we're physiologically wired to eat them. Too many delicious foods are full of carbs, and therefore most of us won't write them off for long. The high protein craze doesn't endure for most because it's not enjoyable. It excludes too many foods people love.

When your self-care is enjoyable to you, it's easy to maintain. Conversely, when it's a "have-to" it's uninspiring. Build your practice and flow zone parameters with activities you like to do and foods you like to eat, or find qualities about these behaviors or foods that are appealing. For example, pick a type of yoga you love or an instructor who has a voice and style you find appealing. Or try that new kale recipe with lots of garlic.

You may be thinking, "How the heck do I make exercise fun or vegetables enjoyable?" Think creatively, think variety, and remember there are unlimited options. There are plenty of healthful foods and a variety of ways to prepare them—at least one of which has to appeal to you. Explore, investigate, experiment, and try new things. Don't be the four-year-old child who has decided she doesn't like carrots so she's never eating anything like them again—including the carrot cake in front of her. You may have written off certain foods or exercises without really trying all your options. Your tastes change as you grow up. It's unlikely you'd choose the same drink at dinner you did when you were seven. Be willing to fall in love with a healthy, fit lifestyle or at least date one.

The next chapter will help you to hone in on the type of movement that will work best for you.

Effective

Your flow zone living must be *effective.* If you're not reaping any benefits from your self-care practice, you're going to get frustrated and want to give it up or go back to extreme measures to reach an outcome.

Are you being effective in your practice? An important thing to remember about the effective ingredient is time. A balance of regular exercise and healthy eating always works to keep a person fit, however it takes time. You may feel the rush of lust from an exciting rendezvous with someone you're extremely attracted to, but the lust doesn't mean the two of you would have a life of happiness together. Immediate results from a fitness program don't always coincide with a long-lasting program. It takes time to build something lasting and valuable, like a good relationship or self-care practice. Instant, superficial results come from extreme programs, and they don't last. Ask yourself if you would rather have a thrilling one-night stand or a rich, long-term relationship? Similarly, would you prefer lasting results via an enjoyable process, or would you choose temporary results brought about by struggle and distress?

How will you know when your self-care is effective? What are your parameters? Define for yourself what you authentically believe to be your markers of success. Will you be exercising regularly? How will you know when you can fire your trainer or shrink? How will you behave, think and feel? What will your body image be? Write it down. (Reference the work you did on your fitness mission statement or goals. This is essentially the same idea.)

Allow time for physical results to appear, and pay attention to how you feel in terms of energy, strength and state of mind. Pay attention to the satisfaction you derive from taking good care of yourself. Give yourself an "atta girl" because the practice of self-care is the goal and you're doing it! It feels really good when you know you're acting in alignment with your meaningful goals or fitness statement. Feeling good about what you're doing, more integrity within, or a sense of spiritual connectedness is what matters.

Effectiveness is a balance between patience and aligned choices. Your experience will be determined by your ability to focus on the essence: how you feel, think about, and act on your self-care. Are you proud of yourself? Have you shifted? Are you feeling and thinking better of your body? Moving it? Fueling it? Listening to it? Dressing your body beautifully right now, not seventeen pounds from now? Remember, the last place you see fitness manifest is in your body. The practice must be present in mind and deed before changes appear in your physique.

Making adjustments to your practice doesn't mean that things have to get harder; it means things will evolve. Your phone is no longer attached to the wall in your kitchen by a spiraled cord; it's mobile. Evolution doesn't mean harder, it simply means growth and new skills. For example, if you've successfully practiced your resonant goal of walking two miles, every day for six weeks, yet your outcome goal of loose jeans hasn't manifested, you may want to change something. You could alter your walking speed, frequency, intensity, or distance. Perhaps you'll want to alternate walking with another form of movement or run your eating habits through the HEED filter. Or perhaps you're so delighted with the walking itself and the fact that you've stuck with it, you're no longer concerned about your pants.

Get used to the idea of varying your routine to continue the effectiveness and entertainment quotient of your self-care. It's so much more fun with a variety of options, and outstanding physical fitness is born of variety. Your mind and body will stop progressing with a stale routine. Change brings growth. Your mind thrives on new information and keeps from deteriorating when challenged or put to learning. Think of all the aspects of life that become better with variety, growth, and change: your wardrobe, culinary repertoire, relationships, career, yard, or technological know-how to name a few. As you continue to take small steps in the ways you move your physical self, you'll keep your body from becoming too efficient at a routine. Additionally, exercise and eating are much more fun and interesting if you stir things up a little.

There are literally millions of resources online and in print to help you mix things up with your physical movement and food selection or recipes. Use your resources.

Whether you build it on goals, self-satisfaction, or the buzz you get from running, your self-care practice should give you results in form or content, tangible or intangible. As you build your practice, remember that variety is the spice of fitness and the leavening of effectiveness. Effectiveness equates to living in the flow zone happily while integrating the essence of what you desire.

Doable

Doable is the best way to describe the final principle to successfully staying in the flow zone. Simply put, your self-care must be physically and mentally possible for you on a daily basis. Baby steps from where you are right now are ideal. Create a practice that's within your capabilities and fits into your life *right now*. You're responsible for building your self-care in a way that brings you success. To do so, it has to fit in to your life today.

So often people decide to set themselves up to fail by choosing an exercise and eating program that's a galaxy away from where they're practicing today. If you have a life already, you won't be able to make a quantum leap with success. Unless, of course you land on a TV show where you have a four-hour training session daily, your food is regulated, and you're shamed weekly with a midriff-bearing weigh-in with a 1,269,340 person audience. That might work *while you're there.*

When it's the busy season at work or you have major family obligations, your eating has to flow with your changing situations and environments. If you have people you need to put your time and energy into, then exercise has to fit in with the human element. When you're on a business trip, you've got to roll with the schedule and eat out daily. Little things such as a gym close to your home or office, fitness videos, or packing healthy snacks can make a big difference in whether or not you stay in the flow zone, especially during busy times. Choose facilities and options that work for your schedule and skill level. Your fitness reality must coincide with the reality of your life, because your body isn't separate from your life.

If you set a course that demands too much of you, you'll give up on it. Remember the emotional jump start and pendulum? If your path involves a huge leap from where you're standing, it will probably be too much for you to manage. You would be wiser to progressively build your self-care one step at a time and make sure it flows with your life today.

⌘ **Mental Fitness Exercise:** Set yourself up to win and keep a healthy self-care practice! Use the HEED filter immediately. Write the principles where you can see them and ask yourself how you can make each situation healthier, more enjoyable, effective, and doable. Feel free to make HEED plans for each environment you function within.

🖱 Go to www.loveyourselffit.com/inspiration for a downloadable version of this exercise.

CHAPTER 18

What's Your Type? Meeting Mr. Routine

"Happily ever after is not a fairy tale. It's a choice."

Fawn Weaver

An essential part of making this self-care thing last, is that you enjoy it. Moving your body and eating healthfully every day are two typically challenging aspects of self-care, but you've got to like what you're doing or you're not going to do it! Performing exercise that doesn't suit you and eating health food you hate are like a date from hell: you're with someone you *really* don't like doing something you *really* don't want to do. Likewise, when you meet a guy you resonate with, time flies and you can't wait to see him again. The same is true with your fitness inspirational type. Once you find your inspirational type, your body LTR will flow smoothly and be a lot more fun.

When it comes to a job or a career, you have the incentive of a paycheck or advancement. In a friendship, you can have an emotional connection, camaraderie, or fun together as a payoff. True love, the integrity of commitment, or the responsibility of children could be what keeps you invested in a marriage. Whatever the reasons, there are usually strong internal motivators or inspiration that keeps you committed to the things you must do every day for long periods of time. You'll want to discover and use these similarly strong motivators for your self-care practice and this is the next step in your falling in love with fitness and practicing it each day.

You maintain things you're committed to (marriage, parenting, or a career) with daily choices. It's not always easy. Your actions may take you away from more enjoyable pursuits, but you choose to take specific actions because of something internal. You do things all day, every day, to keep your commitments and honor your responsibilities. You can use the same authentic values or inspiration that you practice with the other commitments in your life. You can also find your inspirational type.

Effectively motivating yourself comes from understanding yourself and using what you know works to move you into action. When dating, some people use the word "type" to describe a type of person they're attracted to. Some find it helpful to type themselves with exercise as well. There are common themes that inspire people in many areas of life. Fitness is no different. For example, if you love to be involved in a group or won't show up for exercise unless you've made a date with a friend, you could call yourself socially motivated. "I'm a socially motivated type of person—I like to connect with others." Or maybe you enjoy beating the clock, breaking records, or challenging others. "I'm driven by challenge. I like to beat my last performance." Whatever moves you will get you to move!

There are a few outstanding types I've observed over the years. I believe them to be applicable to the majority of people: Hedonist, Competitor, Social Butterfly, Righteous Man, and Zen Master. The following is a quiz to help you determine which inspirational type best suits you. Following the quiz is a description of each type and some ideas about what works best for each.

⌘ **Mental Fitness Exercise:** Take the inspiration quiz to see which type(s) you are.

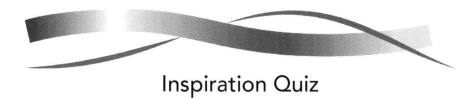

Inspiration Quiz

Decide if the following statements are true or false for you, and give yourself a point for each affirmative answer. At the bottom of the page tabulate your points for each category.

1. _____   I like the "high" feeling I get after a good workout.
2. _____   When I surpass previous efforts I'm elated.
3. _____   I enjoy being with people.
4. _____   There's a right way to do things.
5. _____   I enjoy time to myself.
6. _____   Exercise is more fun with other people.
7. _____   I like to win.
8. _____   I like to be up on the most current research.
9. _____   I have a low tolerance for discomfort, physical or emotional.
10. _____   Silence is heavenly to me.
11. _____   I pride myself on a strong personal compass or sense of what is right.
12. _____   I'm more likely to keep an exercise commitment if another person is expecting me.
13. _____   I like being in the solace of nature.
14. _____   I don't like it when others surpass me.
15. _____   An exercise class sounds like more fun to me than exercising on my own.
16. _____   I enjoy being introspective.
17. _____   I often won't exercise if someone won't participate with me.
18. _____   I believe there are universal principles (moral or logical) of appropriate action.
19. _____   I LOVE food and sometimes eat to discomfort.

20. _____ I sometimes put others ahead of myself.
21. _____ I can't stand feeling sweaty or uncomfortable while exercising.
22. _____ I like being the best at anything I'm involved in.
23. _____ I'm attracted to things that promise a sense of inner calm or peacefulness.
24. _____ I'm more attracted to fun types of exercise, like dance.
25. _____ Competition is appealing to me.
26. _____ I need to believe—see evidence or have a strong inner conviction—before I make a change in my life.
27. _____ I indulge myself sometimes.
28. _____ I will sometimes redo or spend extra time on something until it's done to my satisfaction.
29. _____ Yoga is appealing to me.
30. _____ Sports, games, and competing are more appealing than exercise for its own sake.

Hedonist	# 1, 9, 19, 21, 24, 27	_____ /6 = _____
Competitor	# 2, 7, 14, 22, 25, 30	_____ /6 = _____
Social Butterfly	# 3, 6, 12, 15, 17, 20	_____ /6 = _____
Righteous One	# 4, 8, 11, 18, 26, 28	_____ /6 = _____
Zen Master	# 5, 10, 13, 16, 23, 29	_____ /6 = _____

Consider any category with three or more points a viable motivator for you. The higher the score, the stronger the motivator for you.

Go to www.loveyourselffit.com/inspiration for a downloadable version of these exercises.

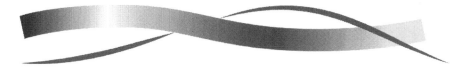

You may have a bit of each inspirational type within you. Identifying your strongest affiliations will help you greatly understand what will motivate you and which types of exercises are good choices for you. The more motivators you can use the better. If you score high in several categories, great! Use as many sources of inspiration as possible.

The Hedonist

The hedonist is a pleasure seeker. We all have a bit of hedonist or we become indulgent at times, but a true hedonist regularly seeks out pleasure or gratification to the point of overindulgence and sometimes detriment. Feeling good physically, emotionally, and mentally are paramount to a hedonist. Hedonists do better with activities and food that are sensory directed or that create positive emotion.

Yoga, Pilates, running, higher-level cardiovascular exercise, fun-oriented activities, dance, swimming, and strength training are all great choices for a hedonist. She generally doesn't like to feel uncomfortable, and therefore requires exercise that can keep her distracted from her own discomfort or activities that give her a "high". (Moisture-wicking and supportive clothing and shoes are a good idea, too.) A fabulous menu is very important. The hedonist doesn't do well feeling deprived, but rather flourishes with a way of eating that looks and feels indulgent. Psychologically, the hedonist will do well to develop self-talk that reminds herself of how good she'll feel after a workout or wise food choice, or how delicious the new recipe will be. *Caution flag:* hedonists tend to be overeaters and under-exercisers. A hedonist would be greatly served by learning how to nurture or reward herself without food (good movie, laughter) and find pleasure in moving her body (sex, massage).

The Competitor

Competitors love a challenge. They want to surpass themselves, beat the stats, or kick the other guy's butt! They expect the maximum from themselves and their bodies. Breaking the record, being the best, scoring, winning, or reaching the goal is vital to the competitor. Comfort is usually secondary. Organized sports, strength training, physical games, using measurements, goals and logs, and any kind of competition or challenge are fantastic motivators for competitors. (A competitor can use numbers *sparingly* if they are truly inspiring.) Eating can be less of an issue, but when it is, the competitor does well to challenge herself to eat better than she did yesterday, make the diet a game, learn about nutrition, or keep a food journal. Psychologically, a competitor only need remind herself of the feeling of winning or reaching her goal to feel a pang of inspiration. *Caution flag:* a competitor can be easily frustrated if she feels there's no chance of a win; she tends toward black-and-white thinking of all or nothing. She's also prone to injuries via not respecting her body's messages or believing the game is more important than her body.

The Social Butterfly

What motivates a social butterfly (SB) are all things social! Interaction with others, talking, and connecting with people are most inviting to a social butterfly. SBs tend to be attracted to fitness that involves others. They do great with personal trainers and coaches, Jazzercise or exercise classes, workout partners, appointments, and general accountability to others. The SB will flourish when she establishes a network of exercise and eating partnerships to keep herself on track. She needs to be mindful of her distraction level while eating. A social butterfly will tend to be more interested in a conversation, a magazine, or a TV program than in listening to her body or paying attention to how she's eating. She'll do great on her healthy eating if several friends or family participate with her.

Caution flag: she'll drop her self-care for another person she perceives to be in need of her assistance or attention. Or she won't show if her partner doesn't. Personal boundaries and self-prioritization are crucial for the SB to learn. She'll tend to put herself last and show up or make goals for others instead of herself.

The Righteous One

The righteous one is someone who believes there's a right way to do things. She has a strong personal belief system. Her convictions can be based in intellect, morals, religion, or personal experience. Either way, discipline to her personal doctrine or beliefs are of utmost importance, sometimes unconsciously. Personal integrity and doing "the right thing" matter most. The righteous one has high expectations and measures herself and others accordingly.

The activities that work best for this type are cross-training (e.g., strength training, cardio, and yoga in a week), periodization program (e.g., following a cyclical strength or cardio training program), martial arts, Iyengar yoga, keeping up on current research, focus on exercise form, and eating "right". She thrives on professional guidance and self-talk which support her personal convictions, as well as reminders and training/eating logs. She who fancies herself a righteous one blooms when she reminds herself of the "right" or important actions she's taken or will take today. *Caution flag:* the righteous one can be too hard on herself, judgmental, or perfectionistic. She can also be too rigid with eating or wear herself out overtraining. Balance, breath work, and laughter are good for her to work in as well.

The Zen Master

A Zen master is partial to all things Zen, especially outdoors. She thrives on a sense of being centered or feeling peacefully content. Escape, quiet, calm, and getting away from the cares, concerns, and stresses of life are extremely attractive to her. She may be introspective or escapist in her sanctuary seeking. Zen masters often prefer to have quiet time to themselves and may get annoyed with chatty partners or instructors. Exercise incentives for a Zen master include nature, the outdoors, time to herself, mind-body modalities, music, and movement that allows time to process thoughts and feelings. Yoga, running, surfing, swimming, snow skiing, individual endurance sports, martial arts, meditation, dance, breath work, and outdoor activities are all excellent choices for a Zen master. Conscious eating is a fabulous path for her, as she gets to immerse herself in the experience of food and eating. She can best inspire herself via her choice of exercise or environment. *Caution flag:* the Zen master can become so enamored with her Zenlike environment or elated state of mind that she neglects to advance or vary her training, or becomes complacent in her efforts or routine. She can also drift away from her self-care practice by getting distracted with other parts of her life.

Dating: Using Your Inspirational Type

As you become clearer about what inspires you, you can talk to yourself about healthier choices. Your mind is the director. For example, if you're a competitor you're motivated by winning. You can tell yourself how wonderful it's going to feel when you beat down your best friend and rival on the tennis court. (Imagine yourself gloating and her crying as you point and laugh and yell "Loser!") If you're a social butterfly you can sign up for or start a healthy cooking group or walking club. (I'm just kidding about the gloating, laughing, "loser" thing. Geez you're ruthless!) If you're a Zen master you love the outdoors, and you can remind yourself of how relaxing it will be when you're away from your desk, at the park, and moving your body through nature. Recall the fresh air, green leaves, sun on your skin, and the like. Feel your motivators and tempt yourself! Talk to yourself. Be your own coach by reminding yourself of what will move you to take action and which things you'll enjoy most about your self-care today. Remember, you're training your puppy-mind, so redirect, praise, repeat. It will help you stay in alignment with your meaningful goals and everyday self-care.

Inspirational-type thinking is actually an exercise aphrodisiac! It will make you randy for your type of movement. "Oh yeah baby, oh, bring me those dumbbells!"

When I started to try exercise regularly, I was a pure hedonist. I valued pleasure and wanted to feel good both physically and emotionally. My hedonistic side made exercise very difficult because it didn't feel good to me. Physically it was uncomfortable because I was heavy, and psychologically it sucked because I felt insecure about my appearance. It wasn't until I discovered running that I found something about it I liked. Running gave me an incredible high. I found out later it's called "runner's high" and boy, did it work for me! Instead of blowing off exercise, I found myself looking forward to it. I realized I was talking myself into exercising. I had found something about running that motivated me: the high. After a run, I felt physically great from the endorphins, and because I had done something healthy I felt emotionally good as well. I would praise myself on my distance or that I ran at all. From that point on, whenever I didn't want to exercise, I would consciously remind myself of how good I was going to feel (how high I'd get) and that was all it took. I was off to the beach or gym in a heartbeat. This is how I discovered my first motivator.

Your motivation will be sparked by exercise you love or through finding something about exercise (or eating healthfully) that strongly appeals to you. It could be other people, competition, the outdoors, time alone, inspiring self-talk, or another gem you discover. Find the personal value in your self-care. Seek out the type of environment, feeling, self-talk, or people (or all of the above) that will move you. Unearth your own inspiration and you'll never need to hire a trainer-sitter, go on another diet, or buy any new fancy gadget to keep you moving. You'll move yourself.

⌘ **Mental Fitness Exercise:** If you haven't done it already, take the inspirational-type quiz and find out what will motivate you. Once you've determined your top motivators, start using the hints and ideas in the description to make a list of all the types of exercise, foods, or healthy adventures you'd like to try. Use the biggest fitness muscle you have—your mind—to inspire yourself to move.

⌘ **Mental Fitness Exercise:** Do-10. Do just ten minutes of exercise in the theme of your strongest motivator(s) ten times. Or try ten different types of exercise that would appeal to your type. You could also try ten different ways to motivate yourself using the suggestions for your strongest type(s).

🖱 Go to www.loveyourselffit.com/inspiration for a downloadable version of these exercises.

CHAPTER 19

Tying the Knot:
Putting It All Together

*"Faith is taking the first step, even when you
don't see the whole staircase."*

Martin Luther King, Jr.

Throughout most of this book the focus has been on internal self-care: the mental, emotional, and spiritual aspects that help or hinder you in finding enjoyable and lasting fitness. This last section is about putting everything you've learned thus far into a workable physical practice.

The majority of programs you've tried in the past may have involved an expert or program that dictated what you should do, eat, and become. As you may know by now, Love Yourself Fit® is a different approach. You're the real director of your self-care practice. You know your strengths and weaknesses, your likes and dislikes, and your inspirations and excuses. No one else wants this for you more than you do. You're the expert on you; therefore you're the best person for the director position.

Designing Your Practice

Putting it all together means taking what you've learned in this book and putting it into a usable, everyday practice. Designing a daily practice then is officially creating your personal treasure map to great self-care.

Imagine it's the day after the proposal from your new fiancé. You've accepted his proposal for marriage, called family and friends, and made passionate love. Now what? Wedding planning aside, the two of you have a new life, commitment, and partnership to define and build together.

The two of you can design your life together any way you'd like: the home you live in, your financial plans, and the manner in which you raise your children. There are an unlimited number of ways for you to build a partnership. You can model yourselves after another couple, listen to advice from friends, read or research topics, seek professional counseling or spiritual guidance, or just wing it, as most of us do, and make up the rules as you go along. Whichever partnership style you choose, both of you have to agree on how things will be handled.

Your daily self-care practice is exactly the same. You can design it any way you'd like. There are plenty of ways to fit fitness into your life. The possibilities are limited only by your knowledge and imagination. You can create, borrow, research, observe, hire, or read about any of the thousands of resources, plans, ideas, gurus, or equipment available to you. You'll find help online, at a library, in a phone call, on TV, radio, DVD, video, at your local YMCA, through a community college or your city's parks and recreation department, at the gym, at a yoga, dance, or martial-arts studio, or at www.loveyourselffit.com. Much may be discovered with just your creativity and a pen. With all these resources, a little imagination, and the things you've learned here, you can create an effective and enjoyable daily practice that suits you perfectly.

The last time you went shopping for jeans, you probably tried on quite a few pairs that didn't fit before you found the best pair. Finding a program or practice that works for you is similar to finding the perfect pair of jeans. While you're shopping for that fabulous fit, you may try on some that are too big or too small and some that are the wrong color or cut. Fitness is the same way. You may have to try on a few programs or practices that don't fit you, are the wrong intensity, or simply don't suit your taste. However, if you invest a little time and thought into tailoring (your practice), you'll get the perfect fit. Keep in mind, you'll probably put less time into designing your practice than you would shopping for those jeans!

At this point, designing your practice will be very simple if you've been doing these:

⌘ **Mental Fitness Exercises throughout the book.** The Mental Fitness Exercises have opened your eyes to your internal blocks and given you the tools to turn them into gravel for your road to fitness. If you have done them, these exercises have directed you to the changes you need to make and taught you how to shift your relationship with your body in a loving direction. If you haven't done them, go back and do so. (Go ahead; I'll wait for you here.) Essentially, the completed mental fitness exercises are your daily practice layout. Assuming you've worked on many of the blocks, used the exercises for you that point to building a daily practice (e.g., sacred time, your meaningful goals, 4-Way Temptation Manager, body gratitude journal, HEED, your inspirational type, etc.), you only have to pull all your results together and down on paper (or screen).

When establishing your practice, start by outlining two or three specific aspects of your self-care on which to focus. You can outline the parameters for your whole self-care practice also, but you may not want to include everything in your life that you want to change immediately. Pick a few core issues to work on initially, and remember that mastery brings confidence for bigger challenges. Baby steps are preferable to galactic leaps.

Get yourself started with a practice you can handle. Try not to set yourself up for failure by committing to a lifestyle light-years away from how you live today. If you're not exercising three days a week now, don't try to launch yourself into a six-day-a-week exercise program. An enjoyable strategy won't push you to extremes by encouraging you to try to lose forty pounds in a month. Once you're consistently exercising three days a week, raise the bar and go for four or five days. Allow the forty pounds to fall off your developing musculature over ten to twelve months and don't sweat measuring it. Releasing a pound of superfluous flesh a week is awesome and easy. Every choice and each day of good self-care will empower and strengthen you. You're building your psycho-emotional muscles as much as you are your mammalian ones. Remember, being fit consists of hundreds of decisions you make all day, every day, over time. You're building Rome here; it may take more than a few weeks.

Use whatever format you prefer: computer screen, stationery, white board, sticky notes, or plain white paper to get your practice outlined. Paint it. Make a collage. Put reminders of it in appropriate places. Make an audio recording and listen to it on your way to work. The form that you choose should be something you enjoy using or looking at daily. What's important is that your practice be made official to you. It's your guide, reference, and inspiration.

Love, Honor, and Obey

When you wed, you make your relationship official. You declare your commitment to the world, your friends, family, the government, and each other. Putting your daily practice in writing makes it official. You can think of committing to your self-care strategy as you would a marriage or partnership agreement. Make a commitment to yourself as you would to your spouse and honor it as you would a marriage.

This certainly isn't necessary, but it is an excuse to buy yourself a pretty ring! If you like, use the following contract to seal your commitment to you.

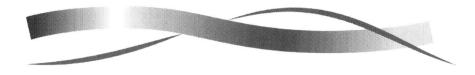

Loving Marriage Contract

Parties Involved: Me and my body
Date and Term: Right now and for the rest of our life
Name of Partnership: _____ (e.g., "Me the Magnificent")

Purpose of Agreement: To create the best possible relationship with each other; love one another to the full extent of our capabilities; nurture inner and physical selves unconditionally; and practice exquisite, enjoyable self-care.

Contributions/Promises/Duties: I agree to: Be loving and nonjudgmental; speak, think, act, and touch body in loving and gentle ways; be understanding and patient of body's progress/schedule for change; listen intently for messages from body; choose the best fuel, movement, and rest possible; remember that psycho-emotional-spiritual-environmental health affects my body and choices; guarantee time (_____ hours/week) to physical and internal self-care.

Body agrees to: Maintain great health and homeostasis to the best of its ability; be understanding of mental-emotional learning curve; continue communication efforts with clear messages; accept loving touch and treatment; be open to new energy, foods, and activities.

Compensation and Benefits: A great relationship with body, fantastic health, flowing fitness, self-confidence and positive body image, healthy relationship with food/eating, enjoyable movement, feel good, total self-love.

Periodic Accounting/Meetings: Parties agree to communicate on a daily basis, with a more thorough meeting every _____ weeks to confirm and ensure progress and satisfaction of both parties.

Forbidden Acts/Prohibitions: Any act of cruelty by either party toward the body or self is not acceptable. This includes mean words; negative judgments; pinching, poking, hitting, or grabbing; abusive intake or outflow behavior; toleration of abusive or cruel commentary, touch, or treatment from others; adoption of "on-off" (arrival) thinking or behavior.

Arbitration Agreement: If either party is dissatisfied with any aspect of the relationship or self-care strategy, terms may be renegotiated at any time. Negotiations must be loving and respectful of both parties' needs and wants.

Signature _____

Date _____

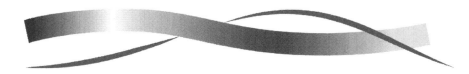

You can make this agreement as official and ceremonious as you wish. Sign it by candlelight, have a witness, or get yourself a ring or whatever else helps make this solid for you.

Allow room in your life and give yourself the space necessary to make your practice a reality. Post reminders, visuals, and affirmations in places you look every day. Let it continually inspire and remind you to love your whole self.

⌘ **Mental Fitness Exercise:** Gather your Mental Fitness Exercises together to outline a daily self-care practice or go to www.loveyourselffit. com/inspiration for a detailed worksheet. Sign the contract if you like, but definitely get yourself a piece of jewelry to make your commitment official!

🖱 Go to www.loveyourselffit.com/inspiration for a downloadable version of the Daily Self-care Practice worksheet.

CHAPTER 20

Marital Therapy: Conflict Resolution

"Happiness can be found, even in the darkest of times,
if one only remembers to turn on the light."

Albus Dumbledore

J ust as you'll have challenges in your career and relationships, initially or periodically, you may have difficult situations arise with your self-care. As with any long-term commitment, you'll have good days and not-so-good days. As in life, expect ebbs and flows. And know there's a way to deal with all the difficult situations that can arise for you. You don't want to camp in the fear of these situations, but knowing how to handle an unexpected upheaval or disturbance when it happens can help you stay in your flow zone.

Build into your self-care practice a Conflict Resolution Strategy (CRS). Be aware of, and prepared for, potential difficulties without diving into the terror of them. For instance, if you have a horrible time eating healthfully at the office, ask yourself how you could better prepare yourself to deal with this environment. Could you alter your office environment by limiting the number of cookies in your cubical or by putting out fresh fruit and nuts instead? Give each of your coworkers a gift of healthy snacks in cute desk-friendly containers so you all can eat better. How about planning days "off" your normal eating to indulge? Can you attend Overeaters Anonymous meetings for support or organize a lunchtime walking group? Plan what you'll need to stay in the flow zone both psychologically and behaviorally.

Eventually, you won't think about these types of environmental alterations. But when you're new at something, for instance parenting or drawing boundaries, it helps to have some tools and to be very conscious of your intentions. Thinking ahead and preparing ways to deal with all kinds of previously "triggery" situations is extremely helpful. Make emergency HEED backup plans for situations you can't control, like your aunt baking a Dutch apple pie while you're visiting. How will you HEED it? Leave and go for a walk? Have a very small piece? Take a piece home and freeze it for one of your days "off". Maybe you'll use your reminders and affirmations, call on your support systems, pray or meditate, listen to a Love Yourself Fit® recording, or use self-talk to get you through the visit feeling good about your choices. Architect a way to implement solutions for life events or times that you know your self-care will be challenged.

Include everyday situations in your CRS. For instance, if you would normally come home after work and use food for reward or comfort, establish a new reward or comfort option. Inevitably, there will be situations that tempt you or throw you off-center; therefore, it's wise to have your CRS in place so you immediately have options and relief. Neglecting to plan for difficult self-care situations is akin to not planning financially for an upcoming mortgage payment or impending retirement. As you become established and the self-care ball is rolling, previously difficult situations won't phase you. Until then, be smart and use the tools you have.

I quit smoking cold turkey by having a CRS in place. I had tried to quit several times before, so I knew which times and places would be the most difficult situations for me, and I built a plan to get myself through those initial tough times. I had a vision of myself as athletic, healthy, and smoke free, which I had based on a friend of mine who was all of the above.

I knew I liked smoking with certain things: coffee, the paper, after dinner, and when going out with friends (Cape Cod = ciggy). These were triggers to my wanting a cigarette. Therefore, when I decided to quit, I planned a strategy to counter these difficult situations. Instead of getting up in the morning to the paper, coffee, and a cigarette, I made a cup of tea and got on an exercise bike. I ate dinner in a different room, read instead of watched TV, and started drinking wine instead of vodka cranberry juice. I changed my daily routine and lifestyle slightly. Mind you, I disliked tea, preferred TV to a book, and at that time hated all wine but the super sweet pink stuff, but I knew they wouldn't trigger me and would make my difficult situations easier. They also fit into my image of what a healthy, fit, non-smoking Lisa would do.

When I quit smoking, I was sharing a house with four other smokers, so I knew the physical cravings would be challenging for me, too. When I wanted to smoke, I did push-ups or crunches, or took a walk outside. I knew from previous attempts to quit that I would have physical withdrawal, and therefore I planned a physical challenge to my cravings: huffing and puffing from exercise. Being out of breath made me want clean lungs instead of a cigarette and again it fit my idea of my desired self-perception. From these tools, my CRS for smoking cessation was born. I kept my eye on the ball throughout, reminding myself of my goal to be free of cigarettes, healthy and fit.

By appropriately planning for the difficult situations I knew I would encounter, I put together a killer strategy that permanently retired my twelve-year, pack-a-day cigarette habit. Sixteen years later I can drink coffee or a Cape Cod without the slightest desire to smoke, and I've come to love tea and bold red wines!

Exploit your past failures and mistakes to develop your CRS. Learn from your shortfalls and misses to alter your strategy for the better. In order to learn from these mistakes, pay attention to what was behind the scenes of errant decisions you've made in the past. What made you stop exercising the last time you gave up? Was it the bubbly step aerobics teacher you found yourself wanting to strangle? Have you previously abandoned commitments when you were feeling bored, frustrated, anxious, or angry? Was your schedule so draining that you couldn't muster the energy to do anything but go home and crash after work? Look for similar patterns in successes and flops. Analyze which situations destroyed your resolve in previous self-care attempts and build a plan to counter them. Put your CRS in writing, too.

Your best CRS will come from incorporating all you know about yourself via past attempts and current issues (needs, beliefs, coping mechanisms, etc.) and also by using your strongest intrinsic motivation, self-talk, and tools to turn difficult situations into peaceful and easy ones. You can do this simply and easily.

Overeating ER!

As part of your marital therapy program or CRS, I would like to introduce you to two body relationship techniques I, and others, have used successfully. The freezer tummy and the 80/20 plan are two of my favorite techniques to use when you're getting started on listening to your body's cues, addressing psycho-emotional aspects of eating, or designing a CRS.

You may recall my mentioning "free days" in regards to eating. Free days are those you relax the "H" in HEED to "h". This means you allow yourself to have the yummy things you normally would have to give up on a traditional diet or lifestyle change. You know the stuff I'm talking about: Brie, French fries, Tres Leches cake, and so on. These foods that may not be nutritionally stellar, but they are delicious and part of life. It's important to honor the enjoyable aspect of HEED by including the foods you love. After all, what is life without the things you love (including double chocolate, bacon-filled donuts)? You can use HEED to stay in the flow zone and find a way to incorporate your favorite foods into your self-care practice.

In order to implement parameters that enable you to work on the psycho-emotional triggers of overeating and learn the physical cues of listening to your body without sabotaging or bingeing, give yourself free days.

I like the 80/20 method. It's an eating guideline that encourages you to eat very healthfully 80% of the time and whatever you want the other 20% of the time. One way to do this is to take weekends "off", or every third day allow yourself a piece of cake or whatever. The 80/20 plan is a good way to curb the food-coping mechanism connection. It's a tool— when you're in the trenches or just starting out—to shrink and control bingeing habits. It's a handy technique for learning to listen to your body. After you've been eating healthy and light for five days and then you don't, you'll feel it! You may feel sick or tired, spacey or just off. Whatever it is for your body, you'll hear what it's saying to you if and when you overeat or eat too much of one thing or another. The 80/20 method is an easy-to-install parameter to help you learn to listen and check your habit while you can get to the bottom of it.

In conjunction, I like to encourage people to use the freezer tummy. What's a freezer tummy you ask? It's your pseudo tummy—the one you fill up with the pizza from softball night or the piece of Dutch apple pie your aunt made. Fill it with anything you want to eat but don't (during your 80% days) and freeze it until your 20% day(s). The concept is so simple your four-year-old will grasp it. Pick up whatever you want to eat, wrap it in a napkin or plastic wrap, and then put it in a gallon freezer bag marked "Tammy's Tummy". It's a beautiful thing, because it eliminates any urgency, deprivation, or fear around food. You won't feel deprived or be afraid you'll miss out; you'll no longer think, "All the yummy lasagna will be gone so I better eat what I can now", or "I really want that, but I can't have it". Yes, you can.

When you put an item in your freezer tummy, an invisible switch flips: "I suddenly don't want sixteen more cookies because they're already in my 'tummy'." It's like a circus trick! I highly recommend it for dining out, holidays, and parties. Your feverish desire to eat everything on the buffet table gets kicked down to a minute urge or disappears all together. I think it's a valuable way to begin to learn to listen to your body or function around a lot of appetizing food while remaining calm. It also enables you to focus on the event or people instead of the food in front of you. Putting the food in the bag and the bag into the freezer is a magic craving eraser. Try it!

You don't have to use the 80/20 plan or the freezer tummy as part of your CRS, but I recommend you integrate something like them. Because when you pull your tummy out of the freezer on Saturday afternoon, you aren't going to want seventy-five percent of the items in that bag. You'll lose the desire to eat most of the things in the bag. They're both tools to help teach you how to better hear your body's communication and simultaneously free you from food bondage.

What if I "Fall off the Wagon"?

You can't! There's no such thing as "falling off the wagon". You'll have ups and downs, but believing that you've "blown it" is to say there's a start and stop point for your body. *There is no "on and off" with your body ever!* Your body doesn't distinguish between Saturday and Monday with different types of digestion or insulin release schedules. It doesn't get the idea of starting over again tomorrow, or that this time, this cookie doesn't count, but yesterday's cookie did. Your body has always been in "on" mode, and always will be—lucky for you!

Besides, thinking that you've failed means you'll start over with the same attack mindset, similar techniques, and another distasteful cycle. Failure means there was a destination to begin with. A process, like life, marriage, or parenting, has no end set point or destination to reach. If you spend every day pining for the end to come, you miss the very point of the experience: being there. Process means being, flowing, evolving, and learning. When you understand that self-care is a lifelong process, you'll recognize that you can't fail.

If you make a poor decision, for instance eating donuts instead of oatmeal, you still haven't blown it. When you think you've failed, you'll tend to excuse the behaviors that follow. How many times after making a bad choice have you said, "Oh well, I blew it! I might as well have another piece and start over tomorrow"? Every day and every choice counts. When you decide you've fallen off your plan or messed up your practice, you're diving into arrival thinking.

Remind yourself that it's not possible to blow it or fall from grace, and affirm that every decision you make can contribute to the next, *better* choice. When you eat ice cream instead of fruit, remind yourself that your next decision is just as important as the last. You're not off until Monday or the first of the month. If you're listening to your body, then one less cookie or bite of ice cream is better than one more. What you intake, how you listen, and the amount you eat always counts. As does the way you speak to yourself before, during, and after you eat, when you look in the mirror, or dress yourself. The amount of exercise you do always adds up. Seven minutes is better than no minutes. Meditating for five minutes will change your entire day for the better. *Everything you do always counts.* All your good choices lead to better health and fitness and build on each other.

If you do fall short of your intentions, go to the source. Figure out what provoked your behavior internally. Drifting out of the flow zone can be a wonderful learning tool and a great opportunity to comb your practice or CRS for weaknesses and shortfalls. What made you choose the ice cream? What were your thoughts? Have you questioned them? Was it an emotional escape attempt? If so, did you try the CORE exercise or something like it? Do you need eating guidelines or better input about this issue? Your relationship with your body won't change or go away by itself. Don't give up or let it slide; *you're worth the effort.* Shift happens!

Every decision and action you've ever taken have collectively brought you to this point in your life. How could you be anywhere else? This is where you need to be to "get it". You need to learn how to take care of yourself from here and now if you expect to maintain your self-care, weight loss, or any other goal. You're right where you need to be to take the next step on your path. Think of yourself not as a work in progress, but a work in *process.* You're the practitioner of your own wellbeing.

I want you to know I struggled a long time with this weight-body issue and never, ever thought I would find a solution. I didn't think there was one out there. I used to ask God why—why did *I* have this problem of overeating and overweight? I thought it was the worst thing in the world as a young female in this body-obsessed culture. And now I see it totally differently. I know now that what I once considered a plague on my life has led me down an incredible path of growth and self-exploration. Without it, I doubt I would have made an effort to be insightful or deal with my psycho-emotional blocks. This issue has given me the opportunity to learn so much about myself and others, relationships, habits, thinking, emotions, spirit, and life in general. I wouldn't now be taking such great care of my body or passing along what I've learned to others.

What if your biggest plague truly is your most tremendous gift? What's this body thing asking you to let go of or forgive? Where's the gift in this for you? See the treasure in your here and now, and turn *your* struggle into your salvation.

Remember, it's hard to fall off the wagon if you're skipping alongside it picking flowers!

⌘ **Mental Fitness Exercise:** Create your CRS from your trigger situations, coping mechanisms, and past failures and use your now overflowing toolbox to build a working CRS. Put it on paper or screen, add it to your daily practice format, and keep it with you.

⌘ **Mental Fitness Exercise:** Make a freezer tummy with your name on it and decide on the 80/20 plan or something similar. Implement all and enjoy!

⌘ **Mental Fitness Exercise:** Ask yourself: in which ways have my issues/ struggle with weight and my body been a gift or helpful for me? What have I learned? How has it enriched my insight, awareness, or personal growth?

🖱 Go to www.loveyourselffit.com/inspiration for a downloadable version of these exercises.

AFTERWORD

A Vision for Your New Life Together

"In everything that moves through the universe, I see my own body and in everything that governs the universe, my own soul."

Chang Tsai

You know now that you're far more than a collection of cells, bones, and organs. When it comes to fitness or weight loss, your belief in the body as a corporeal mass of muscle tissue and digestive processes has faded into the nothingness from which it came. At your core, you are spirit. You've come to know the truth of what true self-care is and where the path to bodily peace begins. It's right here, right now, in thought, feeling, energy, and choice. Intention led by spirit and bolstered by aligned body-mind births a power unstoppable by any measure of baked goods or bacon wrapped fried Brie cubes. You, united, are a force to be reckoned with, a marriage unbreakable.

Fitness, with full reverence for what you are, blossoms to be simple, flowing, easy, and kind. No longer a dreaded pursuit, it emerges a daily practice of love. And you are worth it.

That light-skinned, big-legged Scandinavian girl has grown into a woman with a thriving self-care practice. I still live in sunny southern California, with all those surfer girls. In our forties now, none go bounding down the beach in a bikini, except me. I still don't fit into the beauty box perfectly—there's cellulite under that sarong. This won't stop me. I'm onto the bitch in the mirror; I know her well and her intentions are not my happiness or wellbeing. She hasn't disappeared completely, but we have an understanding—we don't fight anymore. Occasionally, she says something mean and I stick my tongue out at her and remind her she's being a fearful shit again. She's gradually become kinder.

She has to be. There's nothing for us to fight about; there's no more war. We're both on the same team: I'm practicing, peace-filled, and clear. My wish for you is the same.

Reference List

1. J. G. Cannon, "Cytokines in Aging and Muscle Homeostasis," *The Journals of Gerontology Series A: Biological Sciences and Medical Sciences* 50 (1995): 120–23.

2. L. Ferrucci, T. B. Harris;, J. M. Guralnik, R. P. Tracy, M. Corti, H. J. Cohen, B. Pennix, M. Pahor, R. Wallace, and R. J. Havlik, "Serum IL-6 Level and the Development of Disability in Older Persons," *Journal of the American Geriatrics Society* 47 (1999): 639–46.

3. D. Hammerman, "Toward an Understanding of Frailty," *Annals of Internal Medicine* 130 (1999): 945–50.

4. D. R. Taaffe, T. B. Harris, L. Ferrucci, J. Rowe, and T. E. Seeman, "Cross-sectional and Prospective Relationships of Interleukin-6 and C-Reactive Protein with Physical Performance in Elderly Persons: MacArthur Studies of Successful Aging," *The Journals of Gerontology Series A: Biological Sciences and Medical Sciences* 55 (2000): M709–15.

5. Peeke PM, Chrousos GP. Hypercortisolism and Obesity. Annals of the New York Academy of Sciences 1995 Dec 29; 771:665-76

6. Patricia L. Gerbarg and Richard P. Brown, "Yoga: A Breath of Relief for Hurricane Katrina Refugees," *Current Psychiatry Online* 4, no.10 (October 2005) http://www.currentpsychiatry.com/index.php?id=22661&tx_ttnews[tt_news]=169048

7. Evelyn Rubin, "Cosmetics IPO: Highlights from Physicians Formula's S-1 Filing," *Seeking Alpha* (August 28, 2006), http://retail.seekingalpha.com/article/16006.

8. American Society for Aesthetic Plastic Surgery, "Quick Facts: High-lights of the ASAPS 2006 Statistics on Cosmetic Surgery," www.surgery.org/download/2006QFacts.pdf.

9. Ellen Goodstein, "The Basics: 10 Fat Warnings about Diet Products," MSN Money, http://moneycentral.msn.com/content/SavingandDebt/P72445.asp (accessed July 23, 2007).

10. Indiana University Media Relations, "Stick with It! Give Your Workout the Two-Month Test," *Active for Life* (February 14, 2006), http://newsinfo.iu.edu/news/page/normal/2940.html.

11. Michelle Segar, Donna Spruijt-Metz, and Susan Nolen-Hoeksema, "Go Figure? Body-Shape Motives Are Associated with Decreased Physical Activity Participation Among Midlife Women," *Sex Roles* 54, no. 3–4 (February 2006): 175–87.

12. D. G. Rochholz, "Age, Sex, and Socioeconomic Status: Related Factors in Motivation for Exercise," *Sect A: Humanities & Social Sciences* 64, no. 8-A (2004): 282.